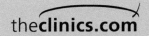

NEUROIMAGING CLINICS

OF NORTH AMERICA

Angioplasty and Stenting for Atherosclerotic Cerebrovascular Disease

Guest Editor
COLIN P. DERDEYN, MD

Consulting Editors
MAURICIO CASTILLO, MD, FACR
SURESH K. MUKHERJI, MD

August 2007 • Volume 17 • Number 3

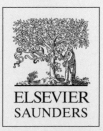

ELSEVIER
SAUNDERS

An imprint of Elsevier, Inc
PHILADELPHIA LONDON TORONTO MONTREAL SYDNEY TOKYO

W.B. SAUNDERS COMPANY

A Division of Elsevier Inc.

1600 John F. Kennedy Boulevard • Suite 1800 • Philadelphia, Pennsylvania 19103-2899

http://www.theclinics.com

NEUROIMAGING CLINICS Volume 17, Number 3
August 2007 ISSN 1052-5149, ISBN-13: 978-1-4160-4336-2, ISBN-10: 1-4160-4336-5

Editor: Lisa Richman

The ideas and opinions expressed in *Neuroimaging Clinics* do not necessarily reflect those of the Publisher. The Publisher does not assume any responsibility for any injury and/or damage to persons or property arising out of or related to any use of the material contained in this periodical. The reader is advised to check the appropriate medical literature and the product information currently provided by the manufacturer of each drug to be administered to verify the dosage, the method and duration of administration, or contraindications. It is the responsibility of the treating physician or other health care professional, relying on independent experience and knowledge of the patient, to determine drug dosages and the best treatment for the patient. Mention of any product in this issue should not be construed as endorsement by the contributors, editors, or the Publisher of the product or manufacturers' claims.

Neuroimaging Clinics (ISSN 1052-5149) is published quarterly by Elsevier Inc., 360 Park Avenue South, New York, NY 10010-1710. Months of issue are February, May, August, and November. Business and editorial offices: 1600 John F. Kennedy Blvd., Suite 1800, Philadelphia, PA 19103-2899. Business and editorial offices: 6277 Sea Harbor Drive, Orlando, FL 32887-4800. Periodicals postage paid at New York, NY, and additional mailing offices. Subscription prices are USD 218 per year for US individuals, USD 336 per year for US institutions, USD 112 per year for US students and residents, USD 252 per year for Canadian individuals, USD 413 per year for Canadian institutions, USD 302 per year for international individuals, USD 413 per year for international institutions and USD 151 per year for Canadian and foreign students and residents. To receive student/resident rate, orders must be accompanied by name of affiliated institution, date of term, and the *signature* of program/residency coordinator on institution letterhead. Orders will be billed at individual rate until proof of status is received. Foreign air speed delivery is included in all *Clinics* subscription prices. All prices are subject to change without notice. POSTMASTER: Send address changes to *Neuroimaging Clinics*, Elsevier Periodicals Customer Service, 6277 Sea Harbor Drive, Orlando, FL 32887-4800. **Customer Service: 1-800-654-2452 (US). From outside of the US, call (+1) 407-345-4000. E-mail: hhspcs@harcourt.com**.

Reprints. For copies of 100 or more, of articles in this publication, please contact the Commercial Reprints Department, Elsevier Inc., 360 Park Avenue South, New York, New York 10010-1710. Tel.: (+1) 212-633-3813; Fax: (+1) 212-462-1935; E-mail: reprints@elsevier.com.

Neuroimaging Clinics is covered by *Excerpta Medica/EMBASE*, the RSNA Index of Imaging Literature, Index Medicus, MEDLINE/MEDLARS, SciSearch, Research Alert, and Neuroscience Citation Index.

Printed in the United States of America.

GOAL STATEMENT

The goal of *Neuroimaging Clinics of North America* is to keep practicing radiologists and radiology residents up to date with current clinical practice in radiology by providing timely articles reviewing the state of the art in patient care.

ACCREDITATION

The *Neuroimaging Clinics of North America* is planned and implemented in accordance with the Essential Areas and Policies of the Accreditation Council for Continuing Medical Education (ACCME) through the joint sponsorship of the University of Virginia School of Medicine and Elsevier. The University of Virginia School of Medicine is accredited by the ACCME to provide continuing medical education for physicians.

The University of Virginia School of Medicine designates this educational activity for a maximum of 60 *AMA PRA Category 1 Credits*™. Physicians should only claim credit commensurate with the extent of their participation in the activity.

The American Medical Association has determined that physicians not licensed in the US who participate in this CME activity are eligible for *AMA PRA Category 1 Credits*™.

Credit can be earned by reading the text material, taking the CME examination online at http://www.theclinics.com/home/cme, and completing the evaluation. After taking the test, you will be required to review any and all incorrect answers. Following completion of the test and evaluation, your credit will be awarded and you may print your certificate.

FACULTY DISCLOSURE/CONFLICT OF INTEREST

The University of Virginia School of Medicine, as an ACCME accredited provider, endorses and strives to comply with the Accreditation Council for Continuing Medical Education (ACCME) Standards of Commercial Support, Commonwealth of Virginia statutes, University of Virginia policies and procedures, and associated federal and private regulations and guidelines on the need for disclosure and monitoring of proprietary and financial interests that may affect the scientific integrity and balance of content delivered in continuing medical education activities under our auspices.

The University of Virginia School of Medicine requires that all CME activities accredited through this institution be developed independently and be scientifically rigorous, balanced and objective in the presentation/discussion of its content, theories and practices.

All authors/editors participating in an accredited CME activity are expected to disclose to the readers relevant financial relationships with commercial entities occurring within the past 12 months (such as grants or research support, employee, consultant, stock holder, member of speakers bureau, etc.). The University of Virginia School of Medicine will employ appropriate mechanisms to resolve potential conflicts of interest to maintain the standards of fair and balanced education to the reader. Questions about specific strategies can be directed to the Office of Continuing Medical Education, University of Virginia School of Medicine, Charlottesville, Virginia.

The authors/editors listed below have identified no professional/financial affiliations for themselves or their spouse/partner:

Allen P. Burke, MD; Mauricio Castillo, MD, FACR (Consulting Editor); Mohamad Chmayssani, MD; Guilherme Dabus, MD; Joanne R. Festa, PhD; Frank D. Kolodgie, PhD; Elena Ladich, MD; Randolph S. Marshall, MD, MS; Christopher J. Moran, MD; Gaku Nakazawa, MD; Lisa Richman (Acquisitions Editor); and Giuseppe Sangiorgi, MD.

The authors listed below have identified the following professional/financial affiliations for themselves or their spouse/partner:

Mark I. Chimowitz, MBChB serves on the advisory committee for M2 Communications.
DeWitte T. Cross, III, MD's spouse is a consultant for Biogen, Berlex, Teva and Amgen; is on the speaker's bureau for Berlex and Tex; and is on the advisory committee for Bio MS.
Colin P. Derdeyn, MD (Guest Editor) is on the Advisory Board for WL Gore and Associates.
Gary R. Duckwiler, MD is a Scientific Advisor for Johnson & Johnson Stroke Management Group, and EV3; and, owns stock in Concentric Medicine.
Yince Loh, MD owns stock in Boston Scientific.
Suresh K. Mukherji, MD (Consulting Editor) is a consultant for Bracco, Bayer, Philips, and Xoran Technologies.
Renu Virmani, MD has research support from Medtronic AVE, Guidant, Abbott, W.L. Gore, General Electric, diaDexus, Takeda, Atrium Medical Corporation, Invatec, ev3, TopSpin Medical (Israel) Ltd., Boston Scientific, NDC Cordis Corporation, Novartis, Paracor Medical, Inc., C.R. Bard, Inc., and Orbus Medical Technologies; is a consultant for Atrium Medical Corporation, Medtronic AVE, Guidant, Abbott Laboratories, W.L. Gore, Terumo, TopSpin Medical (Israel) Ltd., Inflow Diagnostic, Prescient Medical, Cryo Vascular Systems, Inc., and Volcano Therapeutics Inc.

Disclosure of Discussion of non-FDA approved uses for pharmaceutical products and/or medical devices.

The University of Virginia School of Medicine, as an ACCME provider, requires that all authors/editors identify and disclose any "off label" uses for pharmaceutical products and/or for medical devices. The University of Virginia School of Medicine recommends that each reader fully review all the available data on new products or procedures prior to instituting them with patients.

TO ENROLL

To enroll in the Neuroimaging Clinics of North America Continuing Medical Education program, call customer service at 1-800-654-2452 or sign up online at *http://www.theclinics.com/home/cme*. The CME program is available to subscribers for an additional annual fee of USD 175.

ANGIOPLASTY AND STENTING FOR ATHEROSCLEROTIC CEREBROVASCULAR DISEASE

CONSULTING EDITORS

MAURICIO CASTILLO, MD, FACR
Professor and Chief, Division of Neuroradiology, Department of Radiology, University of North Carolina School of Medicine, Chapel Hill, North Carolina

SURESH K. MUKHERJI, MD
Professor and Chief, Neuroradiology and Head and Neck Radiology; Professor, Radiology and Otolaryngology Head and Neck Surgery; and Associate Fellowship Program Director, Department of Radiology, University of Michigan Health System, Ann Arbor, Michigan

GUEST EDITOR

COLIN P. DERDEYN, MD
Associate Professor of Radiology, Neurology, and Neurological Surgery, Washington University School of Medicine, Mallinckrodt Institute of Radiology, St Louis, Missouri

CONTRIBUTORS

ALLEN P. BURKE, MD
CVPath Institute, Incorporated, Gaithersburg, Maryland

MARC I. CHIMOWITZ, MBChB
Professor of Neurology, Emory University School of Medicine, Emory Stroke Program, Atlanta, Georgia

MOHAMAD CHMAYSSANI, MD
Postdoctoral Research Fellow, Department of Neurology, Division of Stroke and Critical Care, Columbia University Medical Center, New York, New York

DEWITTE T. CROSS, III, MD
Associate Professor of Radiology and Neurological Surgery; Director of Interventional Neuroradiology, Barnes-Jewish Hospital and St. Louis Children's Hospital, Washington University School of Medicine, St. Louis, Missouri

GUILHERME DABUS, MD
Division of Interventional Neuroradiology, Gray 241, Massachusetts General Hospital – Harvard Medical School, Boston, Massachusetts

COLIN P. DERDEYN, MD
Associate Professor of Radiology, Neurology, and Neurological Surgery, Washington University School of Medicine, Mallinckrodt Institute of Radiology, St Louis, Missouri

GARY R. DUCKWILER, MD
David Geffen School of Medicine at UCLA, Division of Interventional Neuroradiology, Los Angeles, California

JOANNE R. FESTA, PhD
Assistant Professor of Clinical Neuropsychology, Department of Neurology, Division of Stroke and Critical Care, Columbia University Medical Center, New York, New York

FRANK D. KOLODGIE, PhD
CVPath Institute, Incorporated, Gaithersburg, Maryland

ELENA LADICH, MD
CVPath Institute, Incorporated, Gaithersburg, Maryland

YINCE LOH, MD
David Geffen School of Medicine at UCLA, Division of Interventional Neuroradiology, Los Angeles, California

RANDOLPH S. MARSHALL, MD, MS
Associate Professor of Clinical Neurology,
Department of Neurology, Division of Stroke
and Critical Care, Columbia University Medical
Center, New York, New York

CHRISTOPHER J. MORAN, MD
Professor of Radiology and of Neurological
Surgery, Barnes-Jewish Hospital and St. Louis
Children's Hospital, Washington University
School of Medicine, St. Louis, Missouri

GAKU NAKAZAWA, MD
CVPath Institute, Incorporated, Gaithersburg,
Maryland

GIUSEPPE SANGIORGI, MD
Department of Cardiovascular Diseases,
University of Rome Tor Vergata, Rome; Emo
Centro Cuore Columbus, Milan, Italy

RENU VIRMANI, MD
CVPath Institute, Incorporated, Gaithersburg,
Maryland

ANGIOPLASTY AND STENTING FOR ATHEROSCLEROTIC CEREBROVASCULAR DISEASE

Volume 17 • Number 3 • August 2007

Contents

Frank D. Kolodgie, Gaku Nakazawa, Giuseppe Sangiorgi, Elena Ladich, Allen P. Burke, and Renu Virmani

Atherosclerotic plaque at the carotid bifurcation is the primary cause of ischemic strokes and the degree of carotid stenosis is strongly associated with stroke risk in symptomatic patients. Stroke is the third-leading cause of death in the United States, constituting approximately 700,000 cases each year. In this article, the authors discuss the natural history of carotid and intracranial atherosclerosis, based on their broader knowledge of coronary atherosclerosis. Early to more advanced progressive lesions of the carotid are categorized, based on descriptive morphologic events originally cited for the coronary circulation. The histologic features associated with symptomatic and asymptomatic carotid disease are also addressed, along with the issues surrounding current stent-based therapies for the prevention of major recurrent vascular events.

Colin P. Derdeyn

Atherosclerotic occlusive disease of the cervical and intracranial arteries leads to ischemic stroke through two separate, but interrelated, mechanisms: local thrombosis or embolism from atherosclerotic plaque, and hemodynamic failure (low flow). In this article, the author discusses the evidence linking these two mechanisms with cerebral ischemia, and the evidence for the synergistic effects of thromboembolism and impaired hemodynamics. An understanding of these two mechanisms is important because these mechanisms provide the rationale for revascularization for patients who have atherosclerotic stenosis or occlusion. In addition, the biologic imaging of atherosclerotic plaques and hemodynamic assessment eventually will play an important role in stratifying patient risk and guiding physiologically based patient selection for intervention.

Chronic Ischemia and Neurocognition   313

Mohamad Chmayssani, Joanne R. Festa, and Randolph S. Marshall

Cognitive impairment from a major stroke as a consequence of carotid disease is an acknowledged clinical outcome; however, cognitive impairment without major stroke is open to discussion. The three recognized mechanisms for cognitive dysfunction from internal carotid artery are microembolization, white-matter disease, and hypoperfusion. The last has been most difficult to characterize physiologically. In this article, the authors review evidence supporting the existence of chronic ischemia in the brain and its direct impact on cognitive functions. By incorporating the pathophysiology of chronic ischemia into the algorithm of the management of carotid artery disease, we may be able to extend the goals of carotid artery revascularization beyond merely preventing stroke to include preventing or reversing cognitive decline.

Extracranial Stenosis: Endovascular Treatment   325

Yince Loh and Gary R. Duckwiler

Stroke is the third-leading cause of death in the United States. It occurs in almost 700,000 people per year and cost an estimated $57.9 billion in 2006. Atherosclerotic disease is the cause of one third of these strokes, with more than one half of these stenoses being extracranial in location. Carotid stenoses are usually unifocal and 90% occur within 2 cm of the carotid bulb. Currently, carotid endarterectomy accounts for 117,000 surgical revascularizations per year, whereas carotid angioplasty and stenting are performed less than 10,000 times annually. Stenoses amenable to revascularization are the topic of this article.

Techniques of Carotid Angioplasty and Stenting   337

Christopher J. Moran, DeWitte T. Cross, III, and Colin P. Derdeyn

Carotid angioplasty and stenting (CAS) is an alternative technique to restore a normal lumen for patients who are at high risk for adverse effects with carotid endarterectomy (CEA). CAS has been shown to be of benefit to several groups of patients who have carotid disease and who ordinarily are excluded from many CEA trials. Government payors have approved embolic protection devices (EPDs) and stents for the now reimbursable procedure. In fact, the Centers for Medicare and Medicaid Services are now mandating use of the EPDs in CAS to issue payment. The prudent practitioner will carefully select the patients for CAS with EPD and CEA, so that patients will have the safest opportunity to avoid the devastating effects of cerebrovascular accidents.

Angioplasty and Stenting for Atherosclerotic Intracranial Stenosis: Rationale for a Randomized Clinical Trial   355

Colin P. Derdeyn and Marc I. Chimowitz

Atherosclerotic disease of the major intracranial arteries is a frequent cause of stroke. In addition, many patients who have symptomatic intracranial stenosis are at very high risk for recurrent stroke. Preliminary studies suggest that angioplasty and stenting may reduce the risk of stroke in patients who have severe stenosis of intracranial arteries. Data for angioplasty and stenting, however, consist of case series; no randomized studies have been completed to date. This article reviews these data and discusses the rationale for a randomized trial of angioplasty and stenting versus best medical management for patients who have symptomatic intracranial stenosis.

Dilation of stenoses of the major intracranial arteries is now technically possible in many cases. Using proper precautions, most procedures can be performed without complications today, but the safety margin will likely be improved with refinement of current devices and the introduction of new devices made specifically for this indication. Early experience with these techniques is promising for lowering the risk for recurrent ischemic events in patients who have symptomatic intracranial arterial stenosis refractory to medical therapy. This article describes the steps taken to perform transluminal balloon angioplasty and stent-assisted angioplasty for intracranial atherosclerotic stenosis, from patient preparation through follow-up, including procedural steps and device selection.

Approximately 20% to 40% of patients who have cerebral vascular disease have a vertebral artery–origin stenosis. Atherosclerotic lesions of vertebral arety origin are a potential cause of posterior circulation ischemia, which can be disabling or deadly. Endovascular treatment of vertebral artery–origin and innominate/subclavian artery stenosis has changed in the last 15 years. Surgery usually is successful technically; however, it is also associated with high rates of procedural and periprocedural complications. New techniques and technologies that can be used in the treatment of such lesions are being developed. In this article, the authors discuss the indications, technical aspects, and long-term results of angioplasty and stenting of these vessels.

NEUROIMAGING
CLINICS
OF NORTH AMERICA

Neuroimag Clin N Am 17 (2007) xi

Foreword

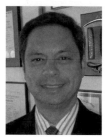
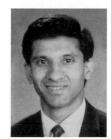

Mauricio Castillo,
MD, FACR

Suresh K. Mukherji,
MD

Consulting Editors

Mauricio Castillo, MD, FACR
Division of Neuroradiology
Department of Radiology
University of North Carolina
School of Medicine Campus
Box 7510
Chapel Hill, NC 27599-7510, USA

E-mail address:
castillo@med.unc.edu

Suresh K. Mukherji, MD
Department of Radiology, B2 A209-0030
University of Michigan Health System
1500 East Medical Center Drive
Ann Arbor, MI 48109-0030, USA

E-mail address:
mukherji@umich.edu

It is obvious to all who practice neuroradiology that treatment of arterial stenoses is becoming an important part of our daily work. The amount of work generated by these patients is much more than just the stenting and includes pre- and postprocedure anatomic and physiologic neuroimaging. Some of this imaging is noninvasive, but other imaging is invasive in nature. To understand the implications of arterial stenting with or without previous balloon dilatation, it is important to understand the basic pathophysiology of the underlying disease as well as patient's symptoms and collateral circulations. This understanding is nicely accomplished in this issue of the *Neuroimaging Clinics of North America* by our guest editor, Dr. Colin Derdeyn, and his collaborators. This issue is divided into four broad sections. The first deals with the pathophysiology of atherosclerotic cerebrovascular disease and contains three articles, including one on the influence of ischemia on cognition. The second section considers extracranial atherosclerotic disease and includes two articles that review endovascular therapies and another that discusses the different techniques available for angioplasty and stenting. The third section of this issue is on intracranial disease. In a fashion similar to the second section, two different articles address the current indications for intracranial angioplasty and stenting and balloon-assisted angioplasty. The content of these two articles is highly technical and should be of interest to vascular surgeons, neurosurgeons, and interventional neurologists as well as to interventional neuroradiologists. The last section is one article on endovascular treatment of the vertebral artery and the innominate/subclavian arteries. As consulting editors, we believe that the topic of cerebrovascular angioplasty and stenting has been covered beautifully by Dr. Derdeyn and his co-authors and congratulate them for this very informative issue of the *Neuroimaging Clinics of North America*.

doi:10.1016/j.nic.2007.05.003
neuroimaging.theclinics.com

NEUROIMAGING CLINICS OF NORTH AMERICA

Neuroimag Clin N Am 17 (2007) xiii–xiv

Preface

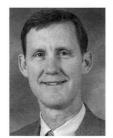

Colin P. Derdeyn, MD
Guest Editor

Colin P. Derdeyn, MD
Washington University School of Medicine
Mallinckrodt Institute of Radiology
Department of Neurology and Neurological Surgery
510 South Kingshighway Blvd.,
St. Louis, MO 63110, USA

E-mail address:
derdeync@wustl.edu

The aim of this collection of articles is to answer the critically important questions of why and how to perform angioplasty and stenting for atherosclerotic cerebrovascular disease. The why is clearly just as important as the how, if not more so. We are treating people, not angiograms. The simple presence of an atherosclerotic lesion is not an indication for a procedure, particularly in the cerebrovasculature.

There is something here for everyone. All readers, including experienced interventionalists, will learn something from the articles on pathophysiology and current indications. This information also will be of use for diagnostic neuroradiologists, neurologists, and neurosurgeons. Interventional neuroradiologists in training and those who have recently graduated will particularly appreciate the articles devoted to techniques.

This issue is organized in four sections. The first section addresses relevant pathophysiology, at both the vascular and neuronal levels. The first article was contributed by Frank Kolodgie, PhD, Associate Director of CVPath, Inc. This company was founded by Renu Virmani, MD, the senior author of the article and formerly the Chair of Cardiovascular Pathology at the Armed Forces Institute of Pathology. She pioneered the techniques for studying the histopathology of stented coronary arteries and is an internationally recognized expert in the biologic responses of the arterial wall to balloon angioplasty and stent implantation. This outstanding article contains information that is critical knowledge for anyone involved in these procedures. I contributed the following article, a review of the mechanisms of stroke related to large artery atherosclerotic disease. Both hemodynamic and embolic mechanisms are involved. This has been an active area of research for my laboratory for more than a decade. The final article was contributed by the group at Columbia University led by Randy Marshall, MD. It is an extremely interesting and important review of the evidence linking hypoperfusion with neuronal reorganization and reduced cognitive function as well as the potential for revascularization to improve cognition. Dr. Marshall's group has been at the vanguard of the active ongoing research in this area. We need to be aware of this line of inquiry: neurocognitive end points are likely to be incorporated in all clinical trials of cerebral revascularization. It is possible that the

doi:10.1016/j.nic.2007.05.002

indications for intervention in the future will be for improvement or protection of cognition rather than for reduction of the risk of stroke.

The remaining sections address the current indications for and technical details of angioplasty and stenting for atherosclerotic stenosis at three specific locations: the extracranial carotid artery bifurcation, the intracranial arteries, and the brachiocephalic/vertebral arteries. The second section focuses on extracranial carotid artery stenosis. Yince Loh, MD, from Gary Duckwiler's group at the University of California-Los Angeles, reviews the accumulating evidence supporting angioplasty and stenting in this surgically accessible segment of artery. Christopher Moran, MD, provides a comprehensive description of the technique of carotid bifurcation angioplasty and stenting, including periprocedural management and the use of distal protection devices. Dr. Moran is a senior interventional neuroradiologist from our team at the Mallinckrodt Institute of Radiology with more than a decade of experience in this procedure. The third section is devoted to the emerging technique of angioplasty and stenting for intracranial stenosis. There is much less literature supporting the use of these techniques in this territory. The first article, contributed by myself and Marc Chimowitz, MBChB, reviews the clinical trials published to date and presents a rationale for a randomized clinical trial. Dr. Chimowitz was the principal investigator for the Warfarin versus Aspirin for Symptomatic Intracranial Stenosis trial, the landmark study of medical treatment for these patients. The second article, by DeWitte Cross, MD, the director of the Interventional Neuroradiology Service at the Mallinckrodt Institute of Radiology, is an in-depth description of the procedural details and technique of intracranial angioplasty. This procedure remains a delicate operation with many opportunities for disaster. The final section is a single article on the indications and technique for angioplasty and stenting of the vertebral origin and brachiocephalic arteries. This article was written by Guilherme Dabus, MD, a skilled interventional neuroradiologist now at Massachusetts General Hospital.

It has been an honor and a pleasure to serve as the guest editor of this issue of the *Neuroimaging Clinics of North America*. I thank Drs. Mukherji and Castillo for their kind invitation to organize this volume. I deeply appreciate the time and effort of the contributors: I owe them one and they know it! I count myself very fortunate for being able to recruit such an outstanding group of clinicians and clinician-scientists. Finally, my thanks go to Lisa Richman and the staff at Elsevier who have been very helpful and supportive.

NEUROIMAGING CLINICS OF NORTH AMERICA

Neuroimag Clin N Am 17 (2007) 285–301

Pathology of Atherosclerosis and Stenting

Frank D. Kolodgie, PhD[a], Gaku Nakazawa, MD[a],
Giuseppe Sangiorgi, MD[b,c], Elena Ladich, MD[a],
Allen P. Burke, MD[a], Renu Virmani, MD[a,*]

- Lesion development at the carotid bifurcation
- Morphologic features of carotid atherosclerosis
- Early nonsymptomatic disease
  Intimal thickening and intimal xanthoma
  Pathologic intimal thickening
- Advanced atherosclerosis
  Fibrous cap atheroma
  Thin fibrous cap atheroma (vulnerable plaque)
- Fibrous cap thickness and lesion instability
- Lesions with thrombi
  Plaque rupture with acute or early organizing luminal thrombi
  Carotid plaque rupture with ulceration

- *Plaque erosion with acute or early organizing luminal thrombi*
- *Nodular calcification*
- Stable atherosclerotic plaque
  Healed rupture/erosions
  Fibrocalcific plaques
  Chronic total occlusions
- The contribution of intraplaque hemorrhage to lesion enlargement instability
- The pathology of bare metal coronary stent implants
- The pathology of coronary drug-eluting stents
- The pathology of carotid stenting
- References

Atherosclerotic plaque at the carotid bifurcation is the primary cause of ischemic strokes and the degree of carotid stenosis is strongly associated with stroke risk in symptomatic patients [1]. Stroke is the third-leading cause of death in the United States, constituting approximately 700,000 cases each year, of which about 500,000 are initial attacks and 200,000 are recurrent. Ischemic stroke accounts for the largest number of new strokes (88%), followed by intracerebral hemorrhage (9%) and subarachnoid hemorrhage (3%) [2]. Histopathologic studies of symptomatic and asymptomatic patients with carotid disease have identified specific lesion characteristics associated with cerebral ischemia, and the underlying mechanisms of plaque instability in the carotid share remarkable similarities with the coronary vasculature [3,4]. In addition to the degree of carotid artery stenosis, the underlying plaque morphology is an important predictor of stroke risk. Intravascular ultrasound and MR imaging studies have shown that echolucent and lipid-rich plaques are associated with plaque rupture [5,6]. In fact, plaque morphology is considered an

[a] CVPath Institute, Incorporated, 19 Firstfield Road, Gaithersburg, MD 20878, USA
[b] Emo Centro Cuore Columbus, via buonarroti 48, 20145 Milan, Italy
[c] Department of Cardiovascular Diseases, University of Rome Tor Vergata, Rome, Italy
* Corresponding author.
E-mail address: rvirmani@cvpath.org (R. Virmani).

doi:10.1016/j.nic.2007.03.006
neuroimaging.theclinics.com

additional independent predictor of cerebral infarction.

In this article, the authors discuss the natural history of carotid and intracranial atherosclerosis, based on their broader knowledge of coronary atherosclerosis. Early to more advanced progressive lesions of the carotid are categorized, based on descriptive morphologic events originally cited for the coronary circulation. The histologic features associated with symptomatic and asymptomatic carotid disease are also addressed, along with the issues surrounding current stent-based therapies for the prevention of major recurrent vascular events.

Lesion development at the carotid bifurcation

The earliest pathologic studies in man described the predilection of atherosclerosis near branch ostia, bifurcations, and bends, suggesting that important components of flow dynamics play an important role in its initiation and development [7]. Atherosclerotic plaque tends to form at regions where flow velocity and shear stress are reduced, in particular at the carotid bifurcation, where disturbances in blood flow deviate from a laminar unidirectional pattern. Plaque burden is greatest on the outer wall of the proximal segment and sinus of the internal carotid artery, in the region of lowest wall shear stress. In marked contrast, the flow divider at the junction of the internal and external carotid arteries, a region exposed to the highest wall shear stress, is protected from atherosclerosis [8]. Thus, the unique geometry and flow properties presented by the carotid bifurcation contribute to the degree and type of atherosclerotic plaque where the underlying morphology often outweighs the actual degree of stenosis, as the most critical determinant of clinical events.

Morphologic features of carotid atherosclerosis

Various plaque morphologies thought responsible for the onset of symptomatic carotid disease have been identified. Because the overall lesion types in the carotid vasculature share the common features of advanced atherosclerosis in coronaries, it seems appropriate that schemes developed to describe the evolution of coronary artery disease may be applied to the carotid, albeit with appropriate modifications. The American Heart Association conventionally uses a numeric classification to stratify various coronary lesion types [9,10]. This scheme, however, implies an orderly, linear pattern of lesion progression, based on the assumption that all

thrombosis occurs from plaque rupture, which later became refuted by the authors' laboratory and others [11–13].

The authors' laboratory subsequently developed a modified classification scheme guided by American Heart Association recommendations, based on the culmination of pathologic findings in more than 200 cases of sudden coronary death (Box 1) [14]. These defined morphologic criteria described for coronary arteries can be applied equally to carotid plaques and may serve as a unifying paradigm to understand the evolution of all atherosclerotic lesions, independent of the vascular bed.

Early nonsymptomatic disease

Intimal thickening and intimal xanthoma

Pre-existing, adaptive intimal thickening and the intimal xanthoma ("fatty streak") are considered the earliest prelesional stage of the disease. Although some human lesions may begin as intimal xanthomas, considerable evidence suggests that the intimal thickening or mass lesion is most likely a precursor to symptomatic coronary disease in humans because these lesions are found in children in similar locations to those of advanced plaques in adults, whereas fatty streaks are know to regress [15]. Histologically, intimal mass lesions consist mainly of smooth muscle cells and proteoglycan matrix, with a variable amount of lipid and little or no surrounding inflammation.

Box 1: **Various lesion morphologies in the carotid artery**

Early nonsymptomatic carotid disease
Diffuse intimal thickening
Intimal xanthoma

Intermediate lesion
Pathologic intimal thickening

Progression of atherosclerosis leading to plaque enlargement
Plaque hemorrhage (± calcification)
Thin cap fibroatheroma (± calcification)

Lesions with thrombi
Plaque rupture with luminal thrombus
Plaque rupture with ulceration
Plaque rupture with organizing thrombus
Plaque erosion
Calcified nodule

Stable atherosclerotic plaque
Healed rupture/erosion
Fibrocalcific plaque
Total occlusion

Pathologic intimal thickening

The transition from an early preatherosclerotic lesion to the more advanced fibroatheroma (defined by a true necrotic core) is marked by an intermediate morphology characterized by extracellular lipid pools within relatively acellular areas rich in proteoglycans [10,14]. The lipid pools tend to develop at sites of adaptive intimal thickening and are located mostly in the deeper intimal layers close to the medial wall, whereas variable numbers of macrophages and T lymphocytes are seen outside the pool, mostly confined to the inner intima (Fig. 1).

Advanced atherosclerosis

Fibrous cap atheroma

The first of the advanced coronary lesions, according to the American Heart Association, is the fibrous cap atheroma [9,14]. The defining feature of this lesion is a lipid-rich necrotic core encapsulated by fibrous tissue (Fig. 2). Fibrous cap atheroma may result in significant luminal narrowing and is also prone to the complications of surface disruption, thrombosis, and calcification. Knowledge of the origin and development of the core is fundamental in understanding the progression of atherosclerotic disease; the question of how lesions convert from lipid-rich pools within pathologic intimal thickening, to plaques with true necrosis (necrotic core), presents one of the most challenging issues in the field today.

Thin fibrous cap atheroma (vulnerable plaque)

Thin-cap fibroatheroma is characterized by a relatively large necrotic core representing about 25% of the plaque area, contained by a thin, fibrous cap defined at less than 65 μm, and heavily infiltrated by macrophages and some T-lymphocytes (Fig. 3) [16]. This well-characterized, ominous plaque is considered the prelude to rupture. The density of macrophages within the fibrous cap is generally very high, although in some cases macrophage infiltration may be less intense and occasionally absent. Because plaque rupture accounts for approximately

Pathologic Intimal Thickening in the Carotid Artery

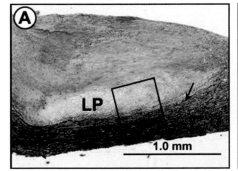
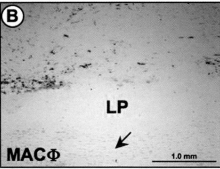
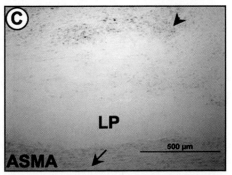

Fig. 1. Pathologic intimal thickening (PIT) in the carotid artery. PITs are considered progressive, early lesions to the more advanced fibroatheroma, or plaques with true necrotic cores. (*A*) Low-power image of an eccentric carotid plaque with a relatively acellular lipid pool (LP) near the medial wall (*arrow*). Note the absence of necrosis. (*B*) Higher-power image representing the region within the black box in *A*, showing an absence of cells within a lipid pool, with surrounding CD-68 positive macrophages (MACΦ) more toward the lumen. (Arrow indicates medial wall.) Infiltration of superficial macrophage into the lipid pool may cause conversion to the more advanced fibroatheroma. (*C*) Anti-α-smooth muscle cell actin (ASMA) immunostaining, showing a distribution of smooth muscle cells (*arrowhead*) more toward the lumen, whereas the lipid pool (LP) is adjacent to the medial wall (*arrow*).

Carotid Artery Fibroatheroma

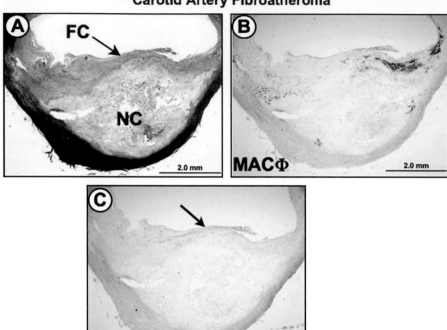

Fig. 2. Serial sections of a carotid artery fibroatheroma. (*A*) Movat pentachrome stain, showing an eccentric plaque with a relatively large necrotic core (NC) covered by a thick fibrous cap (FC). (*B*) A dense region of CD68-positive macrophages (MACΦ) in the shoulder region of the plaque. (*C*) Anti-α-smooth muscle cell actin (ASMA) immunostaining revealing a paucity of smooth muscle cells within the fibrous cap (*arrow*).

75% of thrombi in patients with sudden coronary death, early recognition of thin-cap fibroatheroma is paramount for the identification and treatment of potentially fatal lesions [17]. The thinning or weakening of the fibrous cap leading to fissures and ruptures represents a common mechanism of fibrous cap disruption in coronary and carotid arteries [18]. An interrupted fibrous cap allows circulating cellular and noncellular elements to come in direct contact with the highly thrombogenic components within the necrotic core, and is responsible for luminal thrombosis.

Fibrous cap thickness and lesion instability

It is becoming increasingly clear that fibrous cap thickness and plaque stress are predisposing elements to rupture. In a previous study of sudden coronary death victims, vulnerable plaque was defined histologically, based on a fibrous cap thickness less than 65 μm with regional infiltrates of macrophages (>25 per 0.3-mm–diameter field) [16]. The critical thickness of 65 μm that renders a coronary lesion "vulnerable" is derived from a series of measurements at rupture sites where fibrous caps measured 23 ± 10 μm with 95% of caps 64 μm or less. A similar approach can be

applied to carotid arteries with rupture. In a relatively large series of carotid plaques from the authors' laboratory, the mean fibrous cap thickness was 72 ± 24 μm and vulnerable plaque thickness (95% of ruptured plaques) was identified as less than120 μm (R Virmani, unpublished data, 2007) (see **Fig. 3**). These values are remarkably within the range predicted by flow-plaque interaction models where a fibrous cap thickness of less than 0.1 mm is predicted to induce a large plaque stress that could precipitate rupture, even with an underlying 10% luminal stenosis [19]. In another larger series of more than 412 symptomatic (major stroke or transient ischemic attack [TIA]) and asymptomatic patients who underwent carotid endarterectomy, vulnerable fibrous cap thickness (measured histologically) was defined at less than 165 microns, based on a mean (± SD) cap thickness of 70 ± 47 μm in ruptured plaques (A. Mauriello, G. Sangiorgi, R. Virmani, et al. unpublished data, 2007).

It is the authors' experience that approximately one half of plaque ruptures occur toward the midportion of the cap, rather than the shoulder region, in autopsy plaques derived from sudden coronary deaths. Using a computational finite element model, Cheng and colleagues [20]

Carotid 'Vulnerable' Thin Cap Fibroatheroma

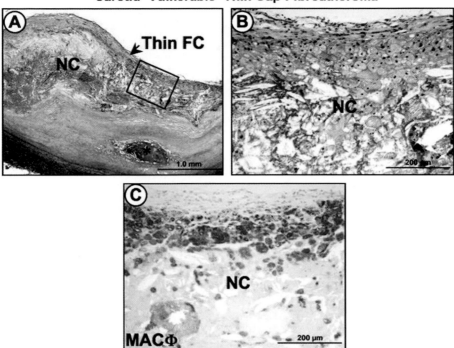

Fig. 3. Thin-cap fibroatheroma "vulnerable" plaque in a carotid endarterectomy specimen. (*A*) Low-power image, showing a carotid plaque with a relatively larger necrotic core (NC) covered by a thin fibrous cap (FC). An area of calcified necrotic core (*) is seen in the deeper intimal layers. (*B*) Higher-power image of an area represented by the black box in *A*, showing the necrotic core and thin fibrous cap infiltrated by foam cells. (*C*) Numerous CD-68 positive macrophages (MACΦ) seen infiltrating the fibrous cap. (*A* and *B*, Movat pentachrome staining.)

calculated the stress distribution in specific coronary artery lesions that caused lethal myocardial infarction and found the average maximum circumferential stress in ruptured plaques was 545 ± 160 kPa. Not all plaque ruptures occurred at the region of highest stress; 10 of 12 lethal lesions ruptured where calculated stress was not maximal, but was 300 kPa. A more precise explanation of why this occurs comes from a more recent study that suggests that minute calcifications of 10-μm – diameter found at sites of relatively high circumferential stress (>300 kPa) in the fibrous cap can intensify the stress levels to nearly 600 kPa when the cap thickness is less than 65 μm [19]. Thus, the site of rupture depends on the relative location, concentrated circumferential stress, and the presence of microscopic calcific inclusions perhaps derived from apoptotic macrophages or smooth muscle cells are present [21]. Collectively, these studies suggest that fibrous cap rupture is very likely a multifactorial event, unpredicted by stress factors or cap thickness alone.

In the coronary arteries of humans, plaque rupture generally occurs in lesions with less than 50% diameter stenosis. The authors' laboratory and others suggest that plaque rupture is not a rare event

in the evolution of coronary atherosclerosis [22,23]. In this context, rupture of the lesion surface is followed by variable amounts of hemorrhage into the plaque, and luminal thrombosis, causing an often clinically silent progression of the disease.

Carotid plaques follow a similar pattern of disruption, with fibrous cap thinning and infiltration of macrophages (see Fig. 3). In a recent study, 47% of ruptured carotid plaque occurred in arterial segments with less than 70% cross-sectional luminal narrowing. Furthermore, a high prevalence of vulnerable plaques occurred in segments not significantly narrowed (80% of cases) (A. Mauriello, unpublished data, 2007). These data suggest that culprit lesions and their precursors occur more frequently in less severely narrowed vessels, and highlight the important tenet that plaques may progress to a substantial size through repeated ruptures before significant luminal stenosis occurs.

Lesions with thrombi

Plaque rupture with acute or early organizing luminal thrombi

Acute thrombosis is characterized predominantly by layered platelet aggregates with variable amounts of fibrin, red blood cells, and acute inflammatory cells. Over time, this provisional matrix heals through a concerted biologic process involving the infiltration of smooth muscle cells, accumulated extracellular matrix proteins (ie, proteoglycans and collagen), neovascularization, inflammation, and luminal surface re-endothelialization.

At least 75% to 80% of sudden coronary deaths show occlusive acute or organized thrombi, and death in the remaining cases is attributed to a "critical" greater than or equal to 75% cross-sectional stenosis in a lesion generally referred to as stable plaque [24]. Although plaque rupture with luminal thrombosis is similarly considered to be the major cause of carotid stroke, thrombi occupying large portions of the lumen in these cases are unusual [3]. The embolic nature of rupture in the carotid is uncharacteristic of coronary plaques because thrombotically active plaques are found in 74% of patients with ipsilateral stroke [4].

Carotid plaque rupture with ulceration

Most pathologists agree that plaque rupture with ulceration is the dominant mechanism that leads to thrombus formation in the carotid disease complicated by embolization and cerebral ischemic events [3,25]. Plaque ulceration is defined as an excavated necrotic core underneath a ruptured fibrous cap, often with large areas of intraplaque hemorrhage and little or no luminal thrombus (Fig. 4). If present, the thrombus is generally small and usually nonocclusive. In a recent large series of carotid endarterectomy specimens from symptomatic and asymptomatic patients that correlated risk factors to plaque morphology, ulcerated lesions were the most common finding, irrespective of clinical status (A. Mauriello, G. Sangiorgi, R. Virmani, et al., unpublished data, 2007). The larger vessel caliber and higher flow velocity of the carotid may explain the embolic nature of these plaques, where shear forces are greater than those of coronary circulation.

Plaque erosion with acute or early organizing luminal thrombi

Plaque erosion is the second-leading cause of acute coronary thrombosis in the coronary circulation. This lesion differs from that of rupture because there is an absence of fibrous cap disruption highlighted by a luminal surface rich in proteoglycans that lacks endothelium. The underlying lesion morphology

Ulcerative Plaque Rupture in the Carotid Artery

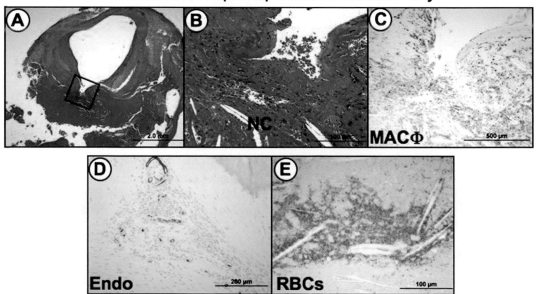

Fig. 4. Serial sections of plaque rupture with ulceration in a carotid endarterectomy specimen. This lesion is the most frequent finding in patients with symptomatic carotid disease. (*A*) Low-power image, showing a disrupted fibrous cap with a relatively large excavated necrotic core (*boxed area*). Note the absence of a significant luminal thrombus. (*B*) Higher-power view of the area represented by the black box in *A*, showing the excavated necrotic core (NC) with recent hemorrhage and cholesterol clefts. (*C*) Numerous CD-68 positive macrophages (MACΦ) seen infiltrating the fibrous cap and surrounding necrotic core. (*D*) Immunostaining with the endothelial (Endo) marker Ulex europaeus lectin, showing intraplaque neovascularization in the plaque shoulder near the necrotic core. (*E*) Old intraplaque hemorrhage in a deep area of the necrotic core rich in free cholesterol (clefts), as visualized by antiglycophorin A immunostaining. (*A* and *B*, hematoxylin and eosin staining.) RBCs, red blood cells.

also differs from rupture because it includes early lesions with pathologic intimal thickening or, to a lesser extent, fibroatheromas without extensive necrotic cores. Erosion is defined as an acute thrombus in direct contact with an intimal surface that lacks endothelial cell coverage. The morphologic characteristics of plaque erosion include an abundance of smooth muscle cells in a proteoglycan matrix and disruption of the surface endothelium without a prominent lipid core [12]. Usually, few or no macrophages or T-lymphocytes are close to the lumen in plaque erosion. Erosions account for approximately 30% to 35% of cases of thrombotic sudden coronary death; they are more common in patients under the age of 50 and represent most of the acute coronary thrombi in premenopausal women [24].

Plaque erosion is an infrequent cause of acute thrombosis in the carotid artery, irrespective of symptoms [3,4]. In the carotid vasculature, the incidence of erosion accounts for less than 10% of all luminal thrombi. It is suspected that the rarity of plaque erosions may be related to the higher flow rates, larger vessel caliber, or relative absence of vasospasm, because erosion in the coronary artery is attributed to episodic arterial contraction and loss of endothelial cells.

Nodular calcification

The "calcified nodule" represents the least frequent cause of luminal thrombus, accounting for 2% to 5% of coronary thrombi [14]. This term is reserved for fibrocalcific plaques with little or no underlying necrotic core, with disruption at the luminal surface and thrombosis attributed to eruptive, dense, calcified nodules. These heavily calcified arteries often show large plates of calcified matrix with surrounding areas of fibrosis, inflammation, and neovascularization (Fig. 5). Although the precise nature of this lesion remains incompletely understood, fragmentation of the calcified plates is believed to be the cause of the nodular calcification, where sometimes even bone formation is seen with interspersed fibrin. Although nodular calcification in deeper regions of the plaque is quite common in the carotid, its association with a luminal thrombus remains infrequent, constituting only 6% to 7% of thrombi (R Virmani, unpublished data, 2007).

Eruptive and Non-Eruptive Calcified Nodules

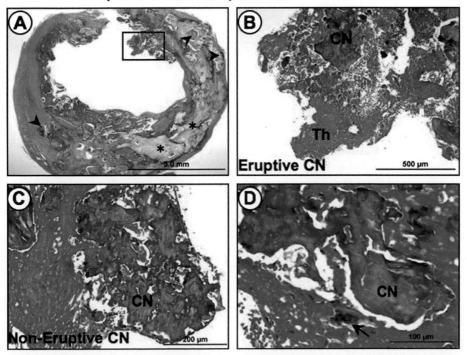

Fig. 5. Eruptive and noneruptive nodular calcification in carotid atherosclerosis. (*A*) Low-power image of a carotid endarterectomy specimen, showing extensive calcification represented by larger plates (**s*) and multiple smaller nodules (*arrowheads*). (*B*) Higher-power image of area represented by the black box in *A*, showing eruptive nodular calcification (CN) with a luminal thrombus (Th). (*C*) Nodular calcification near the luminal surface without a luminal thrombus. (*D*) Higher-power view, showing an osteoclast-like cell, which is frequently associated with nodular calcification. (*A* to *D*, hematoxylin and eosin stains.)

Stable atherosclerotic plaque

Healed rupture/erosions

Healed lesions consisting of previous ruptures, erosions, and total occlusions define a third category of atherosclerotic plaques. Healed plaque rupture in the coronary vasculature is identified based on a disrupted fibrous cap with a surrounding repair reaction [22]. The matrix within the healed fibrous cap generally begins as an early proteoglycan-rich mass, which eventually develops into a collagen-rich scar as the thrombus heals. Healed ruptures frequently exhibit multilayers of necrotic cores with lipid in the deeper intima suggestive of previous thrombotic events contributing to lesion progression [22]. This significant increase in plaque burden and luminal narrowing due to previous thrombosis may occur in the absence of cardiac symptoms. In the authors' series of sudden coronary death patients who died with acute plaque rupture, those with healed myocardial infarction had the highest frequency of healed plaque ruptures [22].

Multiple healed plaque ruptures are also found in the carotid artery and, similarly, a layering of healed repair sites is an underlying cause of luminal narrowing, to some degree. A recent examination of more than 400 carotid endarterectomy specimens shows previous ruptures in approximately 15% of patients (Mauriello, unpublished data, 2007). Although repetitive thrombosis can lead to progressive narrowing in the coronary artery, in the carotid the thrombosis does not typically occupy a large portion of lumen and may explain why multiple healed ruptures are somewhat less prevalent.

Fibrocalcific plaques

Fibrocalcific plaques are lesions recognized by a thick fibrous cap, with an extensive accumulation of calcium typically in the deeper intimal layers [14,26]. These lesions are found frequently in patients with a history of stable angina. Although coronary calcification is highly correlated with plaque burden, its causal relationship in plaque instability is less clear. Because the necrotic core size is usually minimal to absent, this lesion is not considered a true fibroatheroma. Severely narrowed fibrocalcific plaques most likely represent an end-stage, or "burned-out," process of rupture, with healing marked by excessive calcification.

Several mechanisms are likely responsible for calcification of an atherosclerotic plaque, some of which include cell death, expression of selective extracellular matrix proteins, and intraplaque hemorrhage [27,28]. It is unknown whether processes of calcification share similarities with carotid versus coronary lesions or other sites in the vasculature.

In the authors' experience, most lesions from asymptomatic patients who have carotid disease represent fibrocalcific plaques. The frequency of calcification is similar in coronary and carotid arteries, with maximum calcification in carotids occurring in lesions with lumens narrowed more than 70% in cross-sectional area.

Chronic total occlusions

Chronic total occlusions demonstrate varied pathologies, depending on the age of the thrombus [14]. Earlier phases of organizing thrombi are characterized by fibrin, red blood cells, and granulation tissue. Older lesions demonstrate luminal obstruction composed of dense collagen or proteoglycan, with interspersed capillaries, arterioles, smooth muscle cells, and inflammatory cells. Total occlusions often demonstrate shrinkage or negative remodeling of the artery, likely resulting from contraction of the collagen-rich thrombus or extracellular matrix within the plaque. In sudden coronary death victims without a prior history of coronary artery disease, the incidence of total occlusion is 40%, whereas in the carotid, the frequency is much less because the higher flow rates cause most thrombi to embolize.

The contribution of intraplaque hemorrhage to lesion enlargement instability

Recently, the authors' laboratory and others have reported on the significance of hemorrhage as a mechanism of necrotic core enlargement and macrophage infiltration in coronary plaques at autopsy and in the clinic, respectively [29–32]. Red blood cell membranes are an important contributor of cholesterol monohydrate and lipid content in plaques, and leaky vasa vasorum are the most likely source of hemorrhage [32]. Immunostains for glycophorin A (a protein exclusive to red blood cell membranes) are strongly positive in advanced coronary atheroma, whereas early plaques generally show an absence or low expression of glycophorin A. Further, leaky vasa vasorum promote the seepage of extravascular fibrinogen/fibrin, which is observed in 10% to 20% of severely narrowed coronary plaques (R Virmani, unpublished data, 2007). The biologic processes initiated by accumulated fibrinogen/fibrin within an atheroma may constitute an early step in the angiogenic response shared by tumors, wound healing, and inflammation.

Intraplaque hemorrhage is also recognized as an important pathologic process associated with carotid plaque progression and the development of neurologic symptoms, suggesting that hemorrhage itself is related to plaque disruption or may lead to critical stenosis [25,33,34]. The incidence of intraplaque hemorrhage in the carotid circulation is reported to be higher in symptomatic versus asymptomatic patients (84% versus 56%, respectively [3]), and plaque vascularity has been shown to correlate with intraplaque hemorrhage and the presence of symptomatic carotid disease [35]. These new blood vessels could play an active role in the metabolic activity of the plaque and ultimately control the processes that govern plaque progression. In addition, fibrin is a common finding in mature atherosclerotic lesions and most likely represents chronic hemorrhage within the plaque.

The relationship of hemorrhage to necrotic core expansion was demonstrated recently in subjects with carotid atherosclerotic plaques by serial, high-resolution MR imaging. In a prospective study, 154 consecutive asymptomatic patients who had 50% to 79% carotid stenosis detected by ultrasound were evaluated by serial MR imaging every 18 months [31]. In a mean follow-up period of 38.3 months, 12 carotid cerebrovascular events occurred that correlated with carotid MR characteristics of a thin or ruptured fibrous cap, intraplaque hemorrhage, larger intraplaque hemorrhage area, and large necrotic core and plaque dimensions. In another control study of 29 asymptomatic carotid plaques followed over an 18-month period, the identification of intraplaque hemorrhage at baseline was associated with an increased frequency of new hemorrhages and greater enlargement of the necrotic core, when compared with patients without plaque hemorrhage with comparably sized plaques at baseline.

Multiple pathways of entry leading to intraplaque hemorrhage include ruptures/fissures and leaky luminal or adventitial vasa vasorum. Careful study of coronary plaques at autopsy in the authors' laboratory and others suggests that adventitial vasa vasorum are the dominant source of intraplaque neovascularization and hemorrhage [32]. The distribution of adventitial vasa vasorum depends on the vascular bed, and studies have shown that coronary arteries have the largest number of vasa vasorum, followed by carotid, aorta, and renal arteries, with the lowest frequency in femoral arteries [36]. It has been suggested that the extent of vasa vasorum correlates with the rapidity with which atherosclerosis develops in these arteries. This observation is supported further by the fact that vessels that inherently lack vasa vasorum, such as the internal thoracic artery or distal cerebral arteries, also are resistant to the development of atherosclerosis.

Comparative immunohistochemical studies of intracranial and systemic arteries show a relative lack of adventitial vasa vasorum within the intracranial arteries in neonates, children, and adults, although their medial thickness is comparable to their systemic counterparts with vasa vasorum [37]. The existence of vasa vasorum is more common in the proximal arteries (vertebral, internal carotid, and basilar arteries) than in the distal middle cerebral and anterior cerebral arteries [38]. Moreover, vasa vasorum are found more frequently in aged patients who have severe atherosclerosis and in those who have cerebrovascular diseases.

The pathology of bare metal coronary stent implants

After Gruntzig and colleagues [39] originally described the first percutaneous coronary intervention, balloon angioplasty was performed widely for severely narrowed atherosclerotic coronary artery lesions. However, limitations such as high rates of restenosis with early plaque recoil and late arterial shrinkage [40,41] hamper this technique. Compared with conventional balloon angioplasty, the advent of coronary artery stents offers much improved radial strength, thereby preventing acute and chronic causes of narrowing resulting in reduced rates of acute arterial closure and late restenosis [42].

The introduction of stenting, however, was accompanied by a high frequency of acute stent thrombosis, and, despite later improvements in antiplatelet therapy and stent deployment techniques, minor nonocclusive adherent platelet/fibrin thrombi around stent struts are common in early implants of less than 3 days [43]. At 1 month, platelets are no longer apparent, and fibrin usually becomes incorporated into the neointima. Acute inflammatory cells, mainly composed of neutrophils, are associated with stent struts and frequently present in early time periods; however, these cells are rarely observed beyond 1 month [44]. In contrast, chronic inflammatory cells, such as macrophages and giant cells, are present at all time points [44] as a foreign body reaction to the stent itself because the exposure of stent struts is permanent.

From 2 weeks after stent implantation, the neointima consists primarily of smooth muscle cells and proteoglycans. Recognized pathologic factors, such as the degree of medial injury, inflammation, and strut penetration into the necrotic core, are identified as predictors of restenosis resulting from excessive neointimal growth [45]. Moreover, re-endothelialization of the stented luminal surface is considered pivotal, because a deterrent to stent thrombosis and complete endothelialization is typically confirmed by 3 to 4 months in bare metal stents [46,47].

The pathology of coronary drug-eluting stents

Despite the implementation of stent technology over balloon angioplasty, restenosis was still considered a major limitation, with a prevalence approaching 20% to 30% [48]. Because the primary cause of restenosis is excessive smooth muscle cell proliferation, the development of new technologies mainly focused on cell-specific targets aimed at preventing neointimal hyperplasia. The achievements of oral pharmacologic therapy in animal models of in-stent restenosis led to clinical trials in the early 1990s that, for the most part, produced disappointing results [49]. Real clinical success, however, was reached with the advent of localized therapy using stents as the drug-delivery platform [50]. This method of sustained drug delivery takes advantage of polymers to attach and promote controlled elution of drugs from the stent. It was a series of successful preclinical studies [51–54] that paved the way for stent-based local drug delivery in humans.

The first study in humans [55] and the later, larger, multicenter Randomized Study with the Sirolimus-eluting Bx Velocity Balloon-Expandable Stent in the Treatment of Patients with de Novo Native Coronary Artery Lesions (RAVEL) [56] clinical trial produced an astonishing zero percent restenosis.

The local delivery of cytotoxic or cytostatic drugs using a drug-eluting stent (DES) technology has reduced restenosis markedly after percutaneous coronary intervention [57,58]. Currently, polymer-based sirolimus- and paclitaxel-eluting stents are the only DES approved by the Food and Drug Administration and widely used in the United States. Despite the goal of preventing mitogen-induced smooth muscle cell proliferation, the early preclinical studies showed these drugs to delay markedly arterial healing characterized by persistent fibrin deposition and poor luminal surface endothelialization. Further, it is evident from preclinical studies that with continued implant duration comes improved arterial healing with a return of neointimal growth and an absence of long-term effects [51,59].

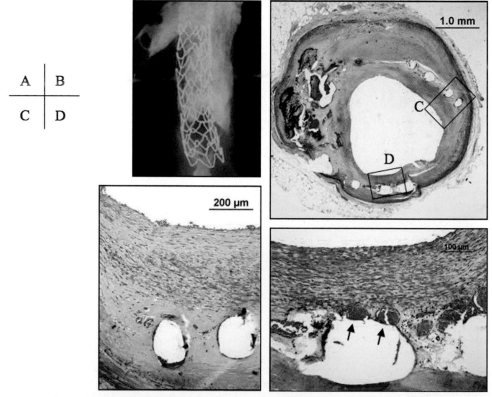

Fig. 6. Bare metal stent in coronary artery at 7 months after implantation. (*A*) Radiograph of the explanted stent, showing severe calcification of the arterial segment evidenced by the hyperdense areas. (*B*) Cross section of middle portion of the stent, showing a widely patent lumen with all struts covered by neointimal growth. (*C*) and (*D*) Higher magnifications of the regions represented by the respective black boxes in *B*, showing a neointima composed primarily of smooth muscle cells and proteoglycans (bluish green on Movat pentachrome) with neo-angiogenesis (*arrows*). (*B* to *D*, Movat pentachrome staining.)

In the emergent age of DES, little was known of their pathologic consequences in humans. The authors' laboratory reported the first histologic findings of a 16-month stent implanted for treatment of an 80% proximal left anterior descending coronary artery occlusion [60]. The device was widely patent, with a minute thrombus at the ostium of a small side branch. Mild neointimal thickening with near-complete healing was evidenced by only little accumulated fibrin near stent struts. Inflammation was rare, and scanning electron microscopy of the luminal surface showed greater than 80% endothelial coverage, with poorly formed endothelial cell junctions and rare platelet aggregates localized to the area of the side branch [60]. At the time, this single stent provided a brief glimpse into the reality of stenting in humans and supported some of the results from earlier animal studies where similar morphologic changes occurred, albeit with a markedly shortened interval of healing. In a later report from the authors' laboratory, they describe a case of hypersensitivity in an 18-month stent implant, which implicates the polymer as the potential culprit for the reaction. Polymers are not all safe [61]. Even in preclinical studies, eosinophilic granulomatous reactions are found around 50% to 70% of stent struts in a 9-month stent implanted in swine coronary arteries (R Virmani, unpublished data, 2007). In the authors' experience, this type of inflammatory reaction has never been observed with bare, stainless steel stents.

A more recent examination of a larger series of DES at autopsy in the authors' laboratory shows early platelet and fibrin thrombi adherent to stent struts, and infiltration of neutrophils, which is fundamentally similar to bare metal stent (BMS) [47]. However, persistent fibrin deposition beyond 1 month was observed frequently in DES, together with chronic inflammatory cells. Moreover, substantial delayed arterial healing with minimal

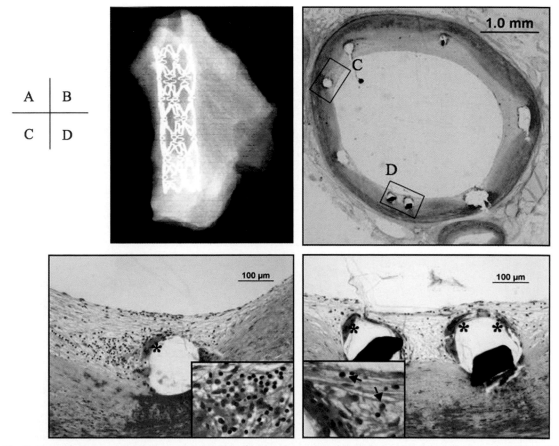

Fig. 7. Drug-eluting coronary stent at 4 months after implantation. (*A*) Radiograph of a well-expanded stent. (*B*) Cross-sectional image, showing minimal neointimal coverage over stent struts. (*C*) and (*D*) Higher magnifications of the regions represented by the respective black boxes in *B*, showing inflammatory cells around stent struts consisting of giant cells (**s*), lymphocytes (*inset in C*), and eosinophils (*inset in D, arrows*). (*B* to *C*, Movat pentachrome stains; insets, hematoxylin and eosin.)

neointimal growth and incomplete coverage of endothelial cells was found consistently in DES cases, regardless of the time after implantation.

In humans, re-endothelialization following BMS implantation in the coronary circulation is near complete by 3 to 4 months, whereas for DES it is projected to take much longer. Moreover, other indications in "real-world" stenting, such as longer lesion lengths, often require overlapping DES, which may further impair re-endothelialization. As a proof-of-concept, the authors implanted overlapping pairs of stents in rabbit iliofemoral arteries, with subsequent en face examination by scanning electron microscopy. These studies demonstrated markedly delayed re-endothelialization at 28 days, in particular at sites of stent overlap, which was persistent up to 90 days after implantation [62].

Recent clinical reports of very late thrombosis occurring in drug-eluting stents beyond 1 year have alerted the medical community to the possible complications of this technology. In the authors' laboratory, the pathologic outcome of the two Food and Drug Administration–approved stents was examined recently in a relatively large series of postmortem cases [47]. Arterial healing, as evidenced by persistence of fibrin, poor neointimal thickening, and incomplete re-endothelialization, was markedly delayed in DES versus BMS, with a mean implant duration of 9 months (Figs. 6–8). Moreover, late stent thrombosis of the target vessel, as defined by more than 30 days, was noted in 14 of 23 patients receiving DES, with 13 patients dying of stent-related causes. Notably, DES with late thrombosis showed an even less matured neointima, compared with patients with DES without thrombotic occlusion. Additional procedural and pathologic risk factors for late stent thrombosis were identified as local hypersensitivity reactions to the stent; ostial or bifurcation stenting; malapposition/incomplete apposition of struts; restenosis; and strut penetration into a necrotic core [47].

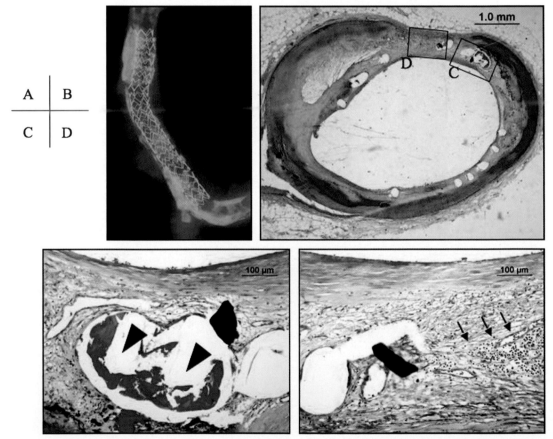

Fig. 8. Drug-eluting coronary stent at 7 months after implantation. (*A*) Radiograph, showing a stent in a tortuous and calcified vessel. (*B*) Cross-sectional image, showing minimal neointimal coverage over stent struts. (*C*) and (*D*) Higher magnifications of the regions represented by the respective black boxes in *B*; note the persistent fibrin accumulated around stent struts (*arrowheads*) together with chronic inflammatory cells of, mainly, lymphocytes (*arrows*).

In DES, re-endothelialization was delayed further, compared with BMS ($55.8 \pm 26.5\%$ versus $89.8 \pm 55.8\%$, $P = .0001$), regardless of implant duration. In fact, BMS had significantly greater endothelialization than DES at all time points studied. How long DES will remain incompletely endothelialized is still unclear. In the RAVEL trial, the neointimal growth increased every year up to the 5-year time point when data are available. As experience grows, our understanding of the pathophysiology of DES, in particular the behavior of endothelial cells, undoubtedly will improve, in particular in devices with longer implant durations.

Recently, the feasibility of DES implantation for intracranial lesions has been studied [63,64]. Although DES showed effectiveness in terms of angiographic results, issues of safety, as noted in coronary arteries, should not be established solely by midterm follow-up. Critical issues, such as vessel tortuosity, calcified lesions, hypersensitivity, and delayed endothelialization, are still unresolved. Moreover, long-term studies are necessary to determine the restenosis rates of DES in cerebral vessels, in particular in comparison with bare metal stents. Finally, the lessons learned from the clinical experience of DES implantation in coronary artery have identified the potential limitation of late stent thrombosis, where the feasibility of a successful antiplatelet regimen should be considered carefully before using an intracranial DES.

The pathology of carotid stenting

The carotid artery is one of the more susceptible locations for atherosclerosis development because its anatomy presents a large bifurcation site with dramatic changes in regional blood flow and shear stresses. Reports of the advantages of carotid endarterectomy over conventional medical therapy led to even asymptomatic patients with severe carotid artery stenosis being treated by this surgical approach [1,65,66]. Many patients however, still remain high-risk surgical candidates because of their comorbidities and, therefore, percutaneous intervention (stenting) for carotid artery stenosis is the current treatment of choice for this population. Recently, Yadav and colleagues [67] reported the favorable results of carotid stenting in high-risk

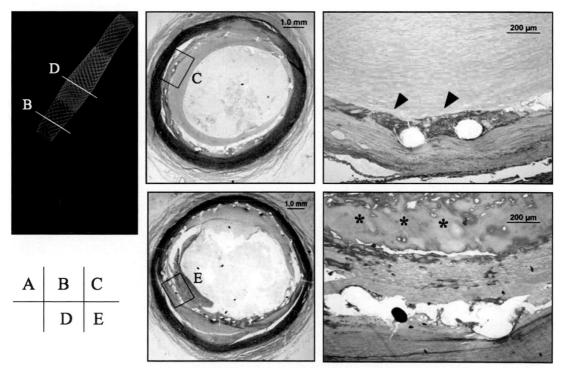

Fig. 9. Carotid artery stent 7 years after implantation. (*A*) Radiograph, showing a pair of similar, overlapping stents with transverse sections taken for histology from the proximal nonoverlap (slice *B*) and middle overlapping (slice *D*) region. (*B*) Cross-sectional image from proximal regions of the stents, showing a widely patent lumen. (*C*) Higher magnification represented by the region within the black box in *B*, showing accumulated fibrin around stent struts (*arrowheads*). (*D*) and (*E*) Low- and higher-power cross-sectional images at a site of strut overlap. Several stent struts remain poorly covered by neointimal growth and are surrounded by a nonocclusive, non–flow-limiting, fibrin-rich thrombus (**s*).

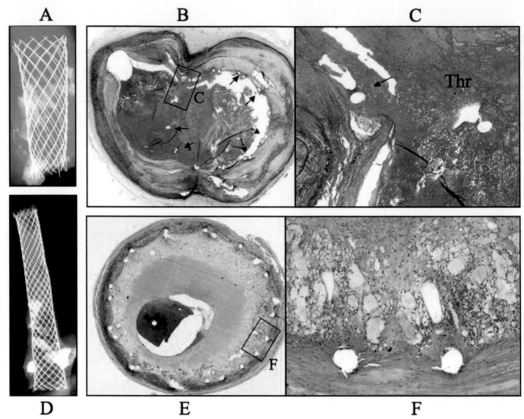

Fig. 10. Carotid artery stents 8 (*A* to *C*) and 10 (*D* to *F*) months after implantation. (*A*) Radiograph of an 8-month stented carotid segment with focal calcification. (*B*) Cross-sectional image at the carotid bifurcation, showing an occlusive thrombus with stent struts remaining uncovered by neointimal growth (*arrows*). (*C*) Higher-power image represented by the area within the black box in *B*, showing a tear in the arterial wall at ostium of side branch (*arrow*) with a superimposed thrombus (Thr). (*D*) Radiographic image of a 10-month carotid stent implant in an arterial segment with focal areas of dense calcification. (*E*) Histologic image, showing severe restenosis with approximately 80% cross-sectional luminal narrowing; a postmortem clot (*) is seen in the lumen. (*F*) Higher-power image within the black box in *E*, showing chronic inflammation and angiogenesis around stent struts.

patients with emboli-protection devices, compared with surgery.

The pathology of carotid artery stents is not well characterized because the tissue availability for study is limited. Comparable lesion morphologies, however, in coronary and carotid arteries are expected to produce similar degrees of healing in response to stenting, although in-stent restenosis after carotid stenting is reported lower, in the range of 4% to 16% [68–70], which may reflect the larger vessel caliber of the carotid. From the authors' small number of autopsy cases, restenosis was documented in those arteries with extensive inflammation. Therefore, persistent inflammation seems an important risk factor of restenosis, which is consistent with coronary stent implants. Anecdotal data suggest that the time course of arterial healing may vary in coronary versus carotid stents. In a recent study by Buhk and colleagues [71], delayed late stent thrombosis (defined as more than 1 week and less than 3 months) occurred in 3 of 96 patients with carotid stenting. In all cases, the postprocedural antiplatelet regimen was discontinued to enable the treatment of a relevant comorbidity. It is possible that re-endothelialization and arterial healing within carotid stents is delayed as a result of high flow rates and the shear forces caused by the bifurcation of carotid arteries. In fact, delayed arterial healing with uncovered struts and persistent fibrin was observed at even later time points among the authors' autopsy cases (Figs. 9 and 10). Further characterization of endothelialization and arterial healing in carotid stents is needed.

References

[1] Rosamond W, Flegal K, Friday G, et al. Heart disease and stroke statistics—2007 update: a report from the American Heart Association Statistics

Committee and Stroke Statistics Subcommittee. Circulation 2007;115:e65–e171.

[2] Thom T, Haase N, Rosamond W, et al. Heart disease and stroke statistics–2006 update: a report from the American Heart Association Statistics Committee and Stroke Statistics Subcommittee. Circulation 2006;113:e85–e151.

[3] Carr S, Farb A, Pearce WH, et al. Atherosclerotic plaque rupture in symptomatic carotid artery stenosis. J Vasc Surg 1996;23:755–65.

[4] Spagnoli LG, Mauriello A, Sangiorgi G, et al. Extracranial thrombotically active carotid plaque as a risk factor for ischemic stroke. JAMA 2004;292:1845–52.

[5] Gronholdt ML, Nordestgaard BG, Schroeder TV, et al. Ultrasonic echolucent carotid plaques predict future strokes. Circulation 2001;104:68–73.

[6] Hatsukami TS, Ross R, Polissar NL, et al. Visualization of fibrous cap thickness and rupture in human atherosclerotic carotid plaque in vivo with high-resolution magnetic resonance imaging. Circulation 2000;102:959–64.

[7] Cheng C, Tempel D, van Haperen R, et al. Atherosclerotic lesion size and vulnerability are determined by patterns of fluid shear stress. Circulation 2006;113:2744–53.

[8] Glagov S, Zarins C, Giddens DP, et al. Hemodynamics and atherosclerosis. Insights and perspectives gained from studies of human arteries. Arch Pathol Lab Med 1988;112:1018–31.

[9] Stary HC, Chandler AB, Dinsmore RE, et al. A definition of advanced types of atherosclerotic lesions and a histological classification of atherosclerosis. A report from the Committee on Vascular Lesions of the Council on Arteriosclerosis, American Heart Association. Circulation 1995;92:1355–74.

[10] Stary HC, Chandler AB, Glagov S, et al. A definition of initial, fatty streak, and intermediate lesions of atherosclerosis. A report from the Committee on Vascular Lesions of the Council on Arteriosclerosis, American Heart Association. Circulation 1994;89:2462–78.

[11] Arbustini E, Grasso M, Diegoli M, et al. Coronary atherosclerotic plaques with and without thrombus in ischemic heart syndromes: a morphologic, immunohistochemical, and biochemical study. Am J Cardiol 1991;68:36B–50B.

[12] Farb A, Burke AP, Tang AL, et al. Coronary plaque erosion without rupture into a lipid core. A frequent cause of coronary thrombosis in sudden coronary death. Circulation 1996;93:1354–63.

[13] van der Wal AC, Becker AE, van der Loos CM, et al. Site of intimal rupture or erosion of thrombosed coronary atherosclerotic plaques is characterized by an inflammatory process irrespective of the dominant plaque morphology. Circulation 1994;89:36–44.

[14] Virmani R, Kolodgie FD, Burke AP, et al. Lessons from sudden coronary death: a comprehensive morphological classification scheme for atherosclerotic lesions. Arterioscler Thromb Vasc Biol 2000;20:1262–75.

[15] Velican C. A dissecting view on the role of the fatty streak in the pathogenesis of human atherosclerosis: culprit or bystander? Med Interne 1981;19:321–37.

[16] Burke AP, Farb A, Malcom GT, et al. Coronary risk factors and plaque morphology in men with coronary disease who died suddenly. N Engl J Med 1997;336:1276–82.

[17] Davies MJ, Thomas AC. Plaque fissuring–the cause of acute myocardial infarction, sudden ischaemic death, and crescendo angina. Br Heart J 1985;53:363–73.

[18] Falk E, Shah PK, Fuster V. Coronary plaque disruption. Circulation 1995;92:657–71.

[19] Li ZY, Howarth SP, Tang T, et al. How critical is fibrous cap thickness to carotid plaque stability? A flow-plaque interaction model. Stroke 2006;37:1195–9.

[20] Cheng GC, Loree HM, Kamm RD, et al. Distribution of circumferential stress in ruptured and stable atherosclerotic lesions. A structural analysis with histopathological correlation. Circulation 1993;87:1179–87.

[21] Vengrenyuk Y, Carlier S, Xanthos S, et al. A hypothesis for vulnerable plaque rupture due to stress-induced debonding around cellular microcalcifications in thin fibrous caps. Proc Natl Acad Sci U S A 2006;103:14678–83.

[22] Burke AP, Kolodgie FD, Farb A, et al. Healed plaque ruptures and sudden coronary death: evidence that subclinical rupture has a role in plaque progression. Circulation 2001;103:934–40.

[23] Mann J, Davies MJ. Mechanisms of progression in native coronary artery disease: role of healed plaque disruption. Heart 1999;82:265–8.

[24] Virmani R, Burke AP, Farb A, et al. Pathology of the vulnerable plaque. J Am Coll Cardiol 2006;47:C13–8.

[25] Avril G, Batt M, Guidoin R, et al. Carotid endarterectomy plaques: correlations of clinical and anatomic findings. Ann Vasc Surg 1991;5:50–4.

[26] Kragel AH, Reddy SG, Wittes JT, et al. Morphometric analysis of the composition of atherosclerotic plaques in the four major epicardial coronary arteries in acute myocardial infarction and in sudden coronary death. Circulation 1989;80:1747–56.

[27] Burke AP, Taylor A, Farb A, et al. Coronary calcification: insights from sudden coronary death victims. Z Kardiol 2000;89(Suppl 2):49–53.

[28] Fischer JW, Steitz SA, Johnson PY, et al. Decorin promotes aortic smooth muscle cell calcification and colocalizes to calcified regions in human atherosclerotic lesions. Arterioscler Thromb Vasc Biol 2004;24:2391–6.

[29] Chu B, Kampschulte A, Ferguson MS, et al. Hemorrhage in the atherosclerotic carotid plaque: a high-resolution MRI study. Stroke 2004;35:1079–84.

[30] Kolodgie FD, Gold HK, Burke AP, et al. Intraplaque hemorrhage and progression of coronary atheroma. N Engl J Med 2003;349:2316–25.

[31] Takaya N, Yuan C, Chu B, et al. Presence of intraplaque hemorrhage stimulates progression of carotid atherosclerotic plaques: a high-resolution magnetic resonance imaging study. Circulation 2005;111:2768–75.

[32] Virmani R, Kolodgie FD, Burke AP, et al. Atherosclerotic plaque progression and vulnerability to rupture: angiogenesis as a source of intraplaque hemorrhage. Arterioscler Thromb Vasc Biol 2005;25:2054–61.

[33] Bornstein NM, Krajewski A, Lewis AJ, et al. Clinical significance of carotid plaque hemorrhage. Arch Neurol 1990;47:958–9.

[34] Imparato AM. The carotid bifurcation plaque–a model for the study of atherosclerosis. J Vasc Surg 1986;3:249–55.

[35] Mofidi R, Crotty TB, McCarthy P, et al. Association between plaque instability, angiogenesis and symptomatic carotid occlusive disease. Br J Surg 2001;88:945–50.

[36] Galili O, Herrmann J, Woodrum J, et al. Adventitial vasa vasorum heterogeneity among different vascular beds. J Vasc Surg 2004;40:529–35.

[37] Aydin F. Do human intracranial arteries lack vasa vasorum? A comparative immunohistochemical study of intracranial and systemic arteries. Acta Neuropathol (Berl) 1998;96:22–8.

[38] Takaba M, Endo S, Kurimoto M, et al. Vasa vasorum of the intracranial arteries. Acta Neurochir (Wien) 1998;140:411–6.

[39] Gruntzig AR, Senning A, Siegenthaler WE. Nonoperative dilatation of coronary-artery stenosis: percutaneous transluminal coronary angioplasty. N Engl J Med 1979;301:61–8.

[40] Mintz GS, Popma JJ, Pichard AD, et al. Arterial remodeling after coronary angioplasty: a serial intravascular ultrasound study. Circulation 1996;94:35–43.

[41] Ryan TJ, Bauman WB, Kennedy JW, et al. Guidelines for percutaneous transluminal coronary angioplasty. A report of the American Heart Association/American College of Cardiology Task Force on Assessment of Diagnostic and Therapeutic Cardiovascular Procedures (Committee on Percutaneous Transluminal Coronary Angioplasty). Circulation 1993;88:2987–3007.

[42] Serruys PW, de Jaegere P, Kiemeneij F, et al. A comparison of balloon-expandable-stent implantation with balloon angioplasty in patients with coronary artery disease. Benestent Study Group. N Engl J Med 1994;331:489–95.

[43] Virmani R, Kolodgie FD, Farb A, et al. Drug eluting stents: are human and animal studies comparable? Heart 2003;89:133–8.

[44] Farb A, Sangiorgi G, Carter AJ, et al. Pathology of acute and chronic coronary stenting in humans. Circulation 1999;99:44–52.

[45] Farb A, Weber DK, Kolodgie FD, et al. Morphological predictors of restenosis after coronary stenting in humans. Circulation 2002;105:2974–80.

[46] Anderson PG, Bajaj RK, Baxley WA, et al. Vascular pathology of balloon-expandable flexible coil stents in humans. J Am Coll Cardiol 1992;19:372–81.

[47] Joner M, Finn AV, Farb A, et al. Pathology of drug-eluting stents in humans: delayed healing and late thrombotic risk. J Am Coll Cardiol 2006;48:193–202.

[48] Kastrati A, Schomig A, Elezi S, et al. Predictive factors of restenosis after coronary stent placement. J Am Coll Cardiol 1997;30:1428–36.

[49] Popma JJ, Califf RM, Topol EJ. Clinical trials of restenosis after coronary angioplasty. Circulation 1991;84:1426–36.

[50] Lincoff AM, Furst JG, Ellis SG, et al. Sustained local delivery of dexamethasone by a novel intravascular eluting stent to prevent restenosis in the porcine coronary injury model. J Am Coll Cardiol 1997;29:808–16.

[51] Carter AJ, Aggarwal M, Kopia GA, et al. Long-term effects of polymer-based, slow-release, sirolimus-eluting stents in a porcine coronary model. Cardiovasc Res 2004;63:617–24.

[52] Drachman DE, Edelman ER, Seifert P, et al. Neointimal thickening after stent delivery of paclitaxel: change in composition and arrest of growth over six months. J Am Coll Cardiol 2000;36:2325–32.

[53] Farb A, Heller PF, Shroff S, et al. Pathological analysis of local delivery of paclitaxel via a polymer-coated stent. Circulation 2001;104:473–9.

[54] Rogers C, Karnovsky MJ, Edelman ER. Inhibition of experimental neointimal hyperplasia and thrombosis depends on the type of vascular injury and the site of drug administration. Circulation 1993;88:1215–21.

[55] Sousa JE, Costa MA, Abizaid A, et al. Lack of neointimal proliferation after implantation of sirolimus-coated stents in human coronary arteries: a quantitative coronary angiography and three-dimensional intravascular ultrasound study. Circulation 2001;103:192–5.

[56] Morice MC, Serruys PW, Sousa JE, et al. A randomized comparison of a sirolimus-eluting stent with a standard stent for coronary revascularization. N Engl J Med 2002;346:1773–80.

[57] Moses JW, Leon MB, Popma JJ, et al. Sirolimus-eluting stents versus standard stents in patients with stenosis in a native coronary artery. N Engl J Med 2003;349:1315–23.

[58] Stone GW, Ellis SG, Cox DA, et al. A polymer-based, paclitaxel-eluting stent in patients with coronary artery disease. N Engl J Med 2004;350:221–31.

[59] Suzuki T, Kopia G, Hayashi S, et al. Stent-based delivery of sirolimus reduces neointimal formation in a porcine coronary model. Circulation 2001;104:1188–93.

[60] Guagliumi G, Farb A, Musumeci G, et al. Images in cardiovascular medicine. Sirolimus-eluting stent implanted in human coronary artery for 16 months: pathological findings. Circulation 2003;107:1340–1.

[61] Virmani R, Guagliumi G, Farb A, et al. Localized hypersensitivity and late coronary thrombosis secondary to a sirolimus-eluting stent: should we be cautious? Circulation 2004;109: 701–5.

[62] Finn AV, Kolodgie FD, Harnek J, et al. Differential response of delayed healing and persistent inflammation at sites of overlapping sirolimus- or paclitaxel-eluting stents. Circulation 2005; 112:270–8.

[63] Abou-Chebl A, Bashir Q, Yadav JS. Drug-eluting stents for the treatment of intracranial atherosclerosis: initial experience and midterm angiographic follow-up. Stroke 2005;36: e165–8.

[64] Gupta R, Al-Ali F, Thomas AJ, et al. Safety, feasibility, and short-term follow-up of drug-eluting stent placement in the intracranial and extracranial circulation. Stroke 2006;37: 2562–6.

[65] Carotid surgery versus medical therapy in asymptomatic carotid stenosis. The CASANOVA Study Group. Stroke 1991;22:1229–35.

[66] Carotid endarterectomy for patients with asymptomatic internal carotid artery stenosis. National Institute of Neurological Disorders and Stroke. J Neurol Sci 1995;129:76–7.

[67] Yadav JS, Wholey MH, Kuntz RE, et al. Stenting and angioplasty with protection in patients at high risk for endarterectomy investigators. Protected carotid-artery stenting versus endarterectomy in high-risk patients. N Engl J Med 2004; 351:1493–501.

[68] Chakhtoura EY, Hobson RW 2nd, Goldstein J, et al. In-stent restenosis after carotid angioplasty-stenting: incidence and management. J Vasc Surg 2001;33:220–5 [discussion: 225–6].

[69] Lal BK, Hobson RW 2nd. Management of carotid restenosis. J Cardiovasc Surg (Torino) 2006;47:153–60.

[70] Wholey MH, Wholey M, Bergeron P, et al. Current global status of carotid artery stent placement. Cathet Cardiovasc Diagn 1998;44:1–6.

[71] Buhk JH, Wellmer A, Knauth M. Late in-stent thrombosis following carotid angioplasty and stenting. Neurology 2006;66:1594–6.

NEUROIMAGING
CLINICS
OF NORTH AMERICA

Neuroimag Clin N Am 17 (2007) 303–311

Mechanisms of Ischemic Stroke Secondary to Large Artery Atherosclerotic Disease

Colin P. Derdeyn, MD

- Cerebral ischemia
- Compensatory mechanisms to low flow
- Thromboembolic mechanisms
- Primary low-flow mechanisms
- Association of low flow and stroke risk
- Synergistic effects of embolic and hemodynamic factors
- Future research directions
- Summary
- References

Atherosclerotic disease of the cervical and intracranial arteries is a frequent cause of stroke. This causality has been established by the frequent association of large artery atherosclerotic (LAA) disease and ischemic events [1,2] and, more importantly, by the benefit of surgical revascularization in large, randomized trials of carotid endarterectomy for patients who had symptomatic extracranial carotid stenosis [3,4] and some subgroups of patients who had asymptomatic stenosis [5]. Likely, both thromboembolic and hemodynamic mechanisms are involved in the pathogenesis of stroke in these patients. In this article, the author reviews the data supporting thromboembolic, hemodynamic, and synergistic mechanisms. An understanding of these mechanisms is important because it is likely that the imaging methods of establishing thromboembolic or hemodynamic risk will become important in identifying patients for intervention, possibly including patients who have asymptomatic atherosclerotic lesions and who are at high risk for future stroke.

The frequency of large artery extracranial or intracranial atherosclerotic disease in patients presenting with transient ischemic attack or stroke varies from study to study, likely owing to racial or environmental factors and study methodology (ie, method of anatomic imaging, if any). Extracranial carotid stenosis or occlusion is among the most common lesions identified in patients presenting with transient ischemic attack or stroke. In a population-based study in Manchester, England, severe carotid stenosis or occlusion was found ipsilateral to the ischemic event in nearly 25% of patients presenting with stroke during a 1-year period [6]. A similar frequency of carotid disease was found in a large series of patients presenting with transient ischemic attack [2]. Intracranial and vertebral-origin lesions are less frequent, accounting for 5% to 10% of patients presenting with stroke [7]. Small-vessel arterial disease and cardiac conditions, such as atrial fibrillation, also account for a large proportion of ischemic stroke.

Cerebral ischemia

Brain tissue requires the continuous delivery of oxygen and glucose to maintain normal neuronal

This article was supported by the National Institute of Neurological Disorders and Stroke, the granting agency, KO8 NS02029 and R01 NS051631.
Washington University School of Medicine, Mallinckrodt Institute of Radiology, 510 South Kingshighway Boulevard, St Louis, MO 63110, USA
E-mail address: derdeync@wustl.edu

doi:10.1016/j.nic.2007.03.001

function. When an artery becomes occluded, the brain supplied by that artery may become ischemic, depending on the adequacy of flow through collateral channels. The cortical surface of the brain often, but not always, has an abundant network of pial collaterals connecting arterial branches. Penetrating arteries into the white matter do not have the benefit of such a network [8]. The survival of brain cells during a period of ischemia is related to several factors. When the delivery of blood to a region of brain tissue falls below a critical threshold, 30 mL of blood per 100 g of tissue per minute in some studies, normal neuronal function ceases. This cessation is related to the reduced delivery of oxygen, not glucose. Glucose is brought into the cells by an active transport mechanism. If flow is restored rapidly, no permanent injury may occur. Irreversible ischemic injury critically depends on both the depth and duration of ischemia [9]. Other factors are also important, including brain temperature, serum glucose levels, and the area of the brain affected. The differential effects on the different components of the neurovascular unit (ie, the neuron, endothelium, and glia) are understood poorly [10]. A thromboembolic stroke often results in a great deal of regional variability in the depth of ischemia. Some ischemic areas may remain viable for up to 24 hours [11]. These regions of ischemic, but viable, tissue have been termed the "ischemic penumbra" [12]. The improved outcome of patients who have been revascularized in the hours after stroke onset has validated this method empirically [13].

Compensatory mechanisms to low flow

Patients who have symptomatic atherosclerotic occlusive disease may have reduced flow to the distal territory, owing to poor sources of collateral flow. Conversely, many patients who have occlusive disease, even complete occlusion, have normal flow, owing to good collateral sources [14]. When perfusion pressure (the difference between mean arterial pressure and the venous backpressure) falls in any arterial territory, the brain and brain vasculature may compensate through two mechanisms (Fig. 1) [15]. The first mechanism is arterial dilation and the second is an increase in the amount of oxygen removed from the blood. Autoregulatory vasodilation is a response by penetrating capacitance arterioles to either reductions in arterial pressure or reduced arterial oxygen content [16,17]. Neuronal, muscular, and physiologic factors are involved in this complex reflex. Arterial resistance is reduced, allowing flow to continue at near-normal rates over a wide range of pressures [18]. Some slight reduction in flow occurs through the autoregulatory

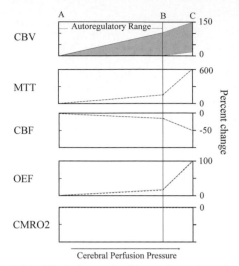

Fig. 1. Modified schematic of hemodynamic and metabolic responses to reductions in cerebral perfusion pressure. The x-axis represents progressive reduction in perfusion pressure. The region between points A and B is the autoregulatory range. The region between points B and C is the region of autoregulatory failure, where cerebral blood flow (CBF) falls passively as a function of pressure. Point C represents the exhaustion of compensatory mechanisms to maintain normal oxygen metabolism, and the onset of true ischemia. Cerebral blood volume (CBV) either remains unchanged or increases with autoregulatory vasodilation, depending largely on the methods used to measure CBV. With autoregulatory failure, most investigators have found further increases in CBV. CBF falls slightly through the autoregulatory range. Once autoregulatory capacity is exceeded, CBF falls passively as a function of pressure, down to 50% of baseline values. Oxygen extraction fraction (OEF) increases slightly with the reductions in CBF through the autoregulatory range. After autoregulatory capacity is exceeded and flow falls upto 50% of baseline, OEF may increase up to 100% from baseline. The cerebral metabolic rate for oxygen consumption (CMRO$_2$) remains unchanged throughout this range of cerebral perfusion pressure (CPP), a reduction owing to both autoregulatory vasodilation and increased OEF. MTT, mean transit time. (*Modified from* Derdeyn CP, et al. Variability of cerebral blood volume and oxygen extraction: stages of cerebral haemodynamic impairment revisited. Brain 2002;125(pt3):603; with permission.)

range [19]. At some threshold point, however, further reductions in pressure exceed the ability of vasodilation to compensate, and flow falls passively as a function of pressure. This situation is known as autoregulatory failure.

The compensatory reflex to reduced blood flow is an increase in tissue oxygen extraction [20,21]. For a given tissue metabolic rate for oxygen consumption, a reduction in the delivery of oxygen (cerebral blood flow) requires an increase in the amount of oxygen extracted by the blood (oxygen extraction fraction [OEF]) [22]. Normal OEF is 30% to 40%, and can increase instantaneously to up to 80%. The precise mechanism by which this increase occurs is not clear. Oxygen is not transported, and reaches the brain tissue by passive diffusion. Tissue oxygen tensions are not reduced when flow falls. It is likely that OEF increases because of a constant flux of oxygen between the tissue and the blood. When flow falls, there is a relative increase in the amount of oxygen used by the brain [23].

In humans, these compensatory mechanisms are identified by several different physiologic imaging methods [14]. Anatomic imaging studies are not sufficient to determine the hemodynamic status in individual patients [24]. Clinical symptoms, with the exception of orthostatic or hemodynamic transient ischemic attacks [25], also are not predictive of hemodynamic status. As a consequence, three broad categories of imaging methods have been developed. Paired flow tests assess the ability of the cerebrovasculature to increase blood flow or blood velocity to a vasodilatory stimulus. If flow fails to increase, pre-existing autoregulatory vasodilation is inferred. Static measurements of cerebral blood flow, blood volume, and mean transit time are another method for identifying the presence of autoregulatory vasodilation. Finally, OEF may be measured directly (Fig. 2). These methods are not interchangeable; different physiologic mechanisms are being assessed. The association between stroke risk and these methods, or the correlation between a candidate method and a proven method, must be proven.

Thromboembolic mechanisms

Thromboembolism from atherosclerotic plaque is the primary mechanism of stroke in most patients who have LAA. The current concept of the vulnerable plaque is accepted widely and is discussed fully elsewhere in this issue. Plaque rupture may lead to platelet aggregation, local thrombosis, or thromboembolism. Plaque material, itself, may embolize [26].

Most of the current knowledge regarding the biology of atherosclerotic plaque and the cascade of events that lead to plaque rupture and platelet aggregation has come from human coronary artery studies and animal models of atherosclerosis. It is likely that these same mechanisms are involved in cerebrovascular atherosclerotic disease. Unlike coronary circulation, local thrombosis is a less common presentation than distal embolism. However, two key differences between coronary and cerebral circulation may make the coronary circulation more vulnerable to local thrombosis and occlusion

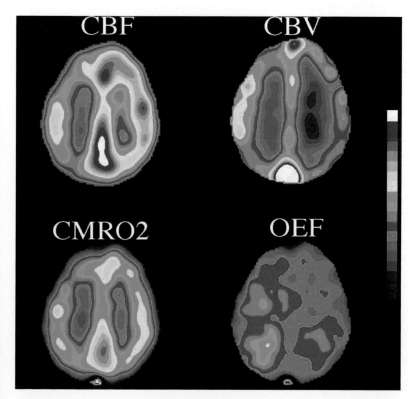

Fig. 2. Positron emission tomography study showing misery perfusion in a patient who has a left internal carotid artery occlusion. Cerebral blood flow (CBF) is reduced, cerebral blood volume (CBV) is increased, and OEF is elevated to compensate for the low flow. Tissue oxygen metabolism (CMRO$_2$) is maintained.

at the site of the atherosclerotic lesion. The first difference is the continuous high flow rate in cerebral circulation. Diastolic flow rates are generally 40% of peak systolic flow. During heart contraction (systole), there is no antegrade coronary artery flow. This episodic stasis may make local thrombotic occlusion more likely to occur. The second factor that may predispose to embolism rather than local occlusion of cerebrovascular vessels is the relatively large vessel diameters of the extracranial vessels, relative to the coronary arteries.

The clinical evidence linking local stenosis to distal embolism is very strong. Platelet thrombi have been observed in retinal vessels distal to atherosclerotic stenoses and have also been identified on surgical specimens after carotid endarterectomy. Single or multiple distal emboli often are identified on angiography in patients who have atherosclerotic carotid disease after acute ischemic stroke [27–30]. Diffusion-weighted imaging in these patients most often shows single or multiple mixed cortical and white matter ischemic lesions, suggesting emboli, even in patients who have clinical lacunar syndromes [31,32]. Finally, embolic events result commonly from symptomatic carotid stenosis. Molloy and Markus [33] monitored the middle cerebral artery for embolic signals using transcranial Doppler (TCD) in patients who had had a recent transient ischemic attack or stroke and severe stenosis of the ipsilateral extracranial carotid artery. Frequent transient high-intensity signals were found in patients who had symptomatic carotid stenosis. No signals were observed in a group of asymptomatic patients who had similar degrees of stenosis.

Primary low-flow mechanisms

Low-flow states are common in patients who have symptomatic LAA [34,35]. When compared with asymptomatic patients who have similar degrees of stenosis, symptomatic patients, as a group, show evidence of hemodynamics impairment (discussed later) [36]. Approximately one half of patients who have complete carotid artery occlusion and prior ischemic symptoms have compensatory mechanisms to low flow in the distal circulation [34]. The presence of hemodynamic impairment in these patients is associated strongly with stroke risk [34,37,38].

Low flow from a proximal atherosclerotic lesion may be an infrequent primary cause of stroke (ie, in the absence of embolism). The association of low-flow states with stroke likely is due to a predisposition to embolic infarction, a synergistic effect of embolic and hemodynamic factors that will be discussed in the next section. The strongest indicator of a hemodynamic mechanism on anatomic

imaging studies is white matter infarctions in the corona radiate or centrum semiovale (Fig. 3) [39–44]. These areas are served by penetrating arterioles from the most distal middle and anterior cerebral arteries and have no potential for collateral supply [8]. This pattern of infarction is associated strongly with underlying hemodynamic impairment [39,40]. It is seen also in situations where thromboembolism may be less likely, such as in patients who have moyamoya phenomenon, cardiac arrest, and global hypotension, or after therapeutic carotid sacrifice. Unfortunately, embolism also may lead to infarction in these brain regions, making this pattern a poor predictor of stroke mechanism [45,46].

Although a hemodynamic mechanism has been implicated clearly in this pattern of infarction, the pathophysiologic factors responsible are unclear. Moody and colleagues [8] performed detailed anatomic studies of these penetrating arteries to the centrum semiovale and adjacent white matter, and found little potential for collateral flow, as opposed to that for the arteries of the pial surface. They hypothesized that these areas, therefore, may be predisposed to a greater risk for ischemia caused by hemodynamic factors than is the overlying cortex. However, researchers in the limited number of neuropathologic studies of acute systemic hypotension consistently have reported white matter injury only

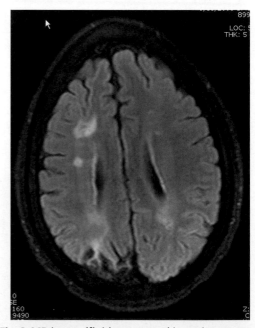

Fig. 3. MR image (fluid-attenuated inversion recovery (FLAIR)) of a patient who has left carotid artery occlusion and increased OEF. In the setting of arterial occlusive disease, lesions in this location are associated strongly with hemodynamic impairment.

in conjunction with infarction of the overlying cortex [47]. In addition, the author has found no evidence for a selective increase in OEF in normal-appearing white matter of the centrum semiovale in patients who have carotid occlusion [48]. This discordance is difficult to resolve.

One hypothesis that may reconcile these data is that collateral flow from the distal anterior or posterior cerebral arteries to the middle cerebral artery (pial collateral vessels) is required for the development of the selective white matter ischemia proposed by Moody and colleagues. Mull and colleagues [49] performed a detailed analysis of the cerebral angiograms of 30 patients who had periventricular white matter infarctions. Eleven of thirteen patients who had unilateral severe occlusive disease of the carotid artery had some restriction of flow across the A1 segment of the anterior cerebral artery. In each of the 11 patients who had A1 segment abnormalities, this restriction was associated with pial collateral flow from the distal branches of the anterior cerebral artery to the middle cerebral artery territory.

In the presence of a normal anterior communicating artery, stenosis or hypoplasia of the A1 segment of the anterior cerebral artery on the side of the occluded carotid artery could result in a greater reduction in perfusion pressure of the middle cerebral artery, relative to the ipsilateral anterior cerebral artery, provided that other sources of collateral flow to the middle cerebral artery (the posterior communicating or the ophthalmic arteries) were inadequate (in terms of maintaining normal perfusion pressure in the middle cerebral artery). The relatively lower pressures in the middle cerebral artery system could lead to the development of pial collateral flow. In this scenario, the pressure in the penetrating arteries to the white matter in the periventricular regions, fed by the most distal branches of the middle cerebral artery that now fill retrograde from small pial collateral channels, may decrease to ischemic levels.

Chronic ischemia is an unlikely cause of infarction to the internal border zone. The author and his colleagues carefully measured OEF in structurally normal white matter of the centrum semiovale in patients who had symptomatic carotid occlusion and found no evidence for higher OEF values in the possible internal border zone compared with OEF values in the cortical and subcortical regions [48]. Selective white matter ischemia may be an acute phenomenon occurring at the time of occlusion that either improves or results in infarction during the time before the positron emission tomography (PET) examination.

The finding of multiple ischemic lesions in a linear pattern in the white matter of the centrum semiovale or corona radiata is associated strongly with severe hemodynamic impairment in patients who have symptomatic carotid occlusion. This association implies a hemodynamic mechanism for this pattern of ischemic injury. Shift of the pial arterial border zone because of reductions of perfusion pressure affecting the middle cerebral artery more than the anterior cerebral artery territory may lead to ischemia of the underlying white matter supplied by penetrating arterioles arising from the most distal middle cerebral artery branches.

Association of low flow and stroke risk

Although hemodynamic or low-flow stroke is unlikely to be a primary cause of stroke in patients who have atherosclerotic disease, strong empiric evidence suggests that hemodynamic impairment is a powerful predictor of stroke risk. Several well-designed prospective studies of hemodynamic status and stroke risk in patients who have LAA have been performed and many have shown a strong association between pre-existing hemodynamic impairment and stroke risk [14]. The strongest associations have been found with measurements of OEF with PET and vasodilatory studies using breath-holding and TCD measurements of blood velocity.

The St. Louis Carotid Occlusion Study was a blinded, prospective study of 81 patients who had symptomatic carotid occlusion, which also specifically assessed the impact of other risk factors [34,50]. The risk of all stroke and ipsilateral ischemic stroke in symptomatic subjects with increased OEF was significantly higher than in those with normal OEF (log rank $P = .005$ and $P = .004$, respectively). Univariate and multivariate analysis of 17 baseline stroke risk factors confirmed the independence of this relationship. The age-adjusted relative risk conferred by hemodynamic failure was 6.0 (95% CI 1.7–21.6) for all stroke and 7.3 (95% CI 1.6–33.4) for ipsilateral ischemic stroke. Similar results were reported in a study by Yamauchi and colleagues [37], using PET measurements of OEF, and by Vernieri and coworkers [38], using breath-holding TCD.

Synergistic effects of embolic and hemodynamic factors

Although low flow is infrequent as a primary cause of stroke in patients who have LAA, it is associated strongly with stroke risk. Several lines of evidence support a synergistic effect of embolic and hemodynamic factors. As mentioned earlier, patients who have symptomatic carotid stenosis, as a group, are much more likely to have impaired vasodilatory responses than asymptomatic patients who have similar degrees of atherosclerotic carotid stenosis. Low flow increases infarct volume in animal models of embolic stroke, and higher baseline flow reduces infarct volume. The clinical features and pattern of stroke in patients who have LAA and hemodynamic impairment are most consistent with embolic mechanisms [32]. It is likely that pre-existing hemodynamic impairment predisposes to ischemic stroke in patients who have an embologenic atherosclerotic lesion.

Asymptomatic emboli are common in patients who have symptomatic carotid disease [33]. Some evidence from animal and human studies suggests a synergistic effect between pre-existing hemodynamic impairment and embolic injury, creating a larger area of infarction than might occur with embolism alone. Omae and colleagues [51] ligated the common carotid artery in a group of experimental rats. Common carotid artery ligation in the rat is a reproducible model of temporary hemodynamic impairment, without causing infarction [52]. Over time, generally within a month, hemodynamics normalize as collateral channels increase in size to accommodate increased flow [53]. The external carotid artery was then retrograde cannulated in the experimental group and in a group of animals with a patent common carotid artery. Two thousand 50-um microspheres then were injected through the external to internal carotid catheter to simulate an embolic shower. The occlusion group had significantly larger infarctions and greater deficits, by functional outcome measures. A second line of evidence supporting this hypothesis is the finding that increased basal cerebral blood flow reduces infarction size in models of temporary middle cerebral artery occlusion [54]. Finally, Pullicino and co-workers [55] found that patients who had low cardiac ejection fraction (<35%) and severe carotid artery stenosis had larger volumes of cerebral infarction than patients who had similar carotid disease and normal ejection fraction.

The author and his colleagues performed a retrospective analysis of the clinical and imaging features of stroke in patients who had known, pre-existing, severe hemodynamic impairment. These patients had symptomatic carotid occlusion and had increased OEF in the distal hemisphere, as measured with PET. They were enrolled in a longitudinal study of hemodynamics and stroke risk. Eleven patients experienced a stroke during the follow-up period of this study. Most were classic thromboembolic events, occurring in core middle cortery territory, involving the cortex and underlying white matter. These data support the hypothesis of a synergistic effect of hemodynamic and embolic mechanisms.

Patients who have pre-existing hemodynamic failure may be at greater risk for a clinical stroke after a thromboembolic event through several mechanisms. Grubb and colleagues [34] suggested that either hemodynamic failure predisposes to the formation of thromboemboli, or thromboemboli may cause infarction more readily in the setting of poor collateral circulation. The later theory was advanced further by Caplan and Hennerici [56], who suggested that hemodynamic failure may lead to delayed washout of microembolic material [34,56].

Future research directions

The development of molecular imaging methods and tools of hemodynamic assessment have great potential to advance our knowledge of stroke risk in patients who have atherosclerotic occlusive disease. In addition, the ability to identify subgroups of patients with higher or lower natural history risks may allow us to address more specific therapies and improve patient outcome. At present, the primary criteria for determining eligibility for intervention are primitive (ie, the degree of stenosis and the presence or absence of ischemic symptoms). These criteria are likely surrogate markers of either unstable plaque biology, hemodynamic impairment, or both. The ability to identify at-risk plaque or hemodynamic impairment may allow the development of therapies targeted at the underlying pathology.

For example, patients who have asymptomatic extracranial carotid stenosis, as a group, have a low risk for future stroke on medical therapy. Carotid endarterectomy provides a benefit for relatively healthy men, but not women. This benefit is marginal, a 1% annual absolute risk reduction. Patient selection is based primarily on the degree of stenosis. Angioplasty and stenting has not been shown to be effective. Emerging evidence suggests that hemodynamic status is a strong predictor of future stroke in these patients.

Silvestrini and colleagues performed a longitudinal study of 95 asymptomatic patients who had greater than 70% carotid artery stenosis [57]. At study enrollment, measurements of middle cerebral artery mean flow velocity were acquired at baseline and after 30 seconds of breath-holding. Patients who had hemodynamic impairment, defined as a reduced or absent elevation in velocity (as compared with normal controls), were at a much higher risk for future stroke than asymptomatic patients who had normal vasodilatory flow responses. Molloy and colleagues performed a similar study using TCD to identify silent embolic events [33]. Patients who had silent emboli had a much higher risk for future stroke.

Randomized studies of endarterectomy or angioplasty and stenting should be pursued in these patient populations found to be at high risk for stroke based on hemodynamic or plaque-specific thromboembolic factors. Patient populations that should be targeted are those at high surgical risk for endarterectomy (ie, no current proven effective therapy), which would include women, patients with prior surgery or neck irradiation, and those with surgically inaccessible lesions.

An example of the use of biologic imaging to identify high-risk subgroups is the Carotid Occlusion Surgery Study (COSS). Increased OEF is a proven, independent predictor of stroke risk in patients who have symptomatic complete carotid occlusion. A regional increase in OEF distal to the occluded carotid artery is present in up to 50% of these patients. No proven effective therapy reduces stroke risk in this population. The extracranial (EC) to intracranial (IC) bypass trial failed to show a benefit when applied to an unselected group of patients who had symptomatic atherosclerotic carotid occlusion, but may have failed because of the inclusion of a large group of patients with little to gain from another source of collateral flow. In the COSS trial, patients are screened with PET for increased OEF. Eligible patients are randomized to surgery or best medical therapy.

Summary

In conclusion, the mechanism of stroke in patients who have atherosclerotic occlusive disease of the carotid artery and its intracranial branches includes both thromboembolic and hemodynamic mechanisms. Either may occur in isolation, but most strokes likely represent a synergistic effect of both mechanisms. In the future, identification of hemodynamic and thromboembolic risk factors will play an important role in selecting patients for medical or endovascular intervention, based on differential natural history risks owing to the underlying physiology.

References

[1] Mead GE, Shingler H, Farrell A, et al. Carotid disease in acute stroke. Age Ageing 1998;27(6): 677–82.

[2] Bogousslavsky J, Hachinski VC, Boughner DR, et al. Cardiac and arterial lesions in transient ischemic attacks. Arch Neurol 1986;43:223–8.

[3] North American Symptomatic Carotid Endarterectomy Trial (NASCET) Collaborators. Beneficial effect of carotid endarterectomy in symptomatic patients with high-grade carotid stenosis. N Engl J Med 1991;325:445–53.

[4] European Carotid Surgery Trialists' Collaborative Group. MRC European Carotid Surgery Trial: interim results for symptomatic patients with severe (70–99%) or with mild (0–29%) carotid stenosis. Lancet 1991;337:1235–43.

[5] Executive Committee of the Asymptomatic Carotid Atherosclerosis Study. Endarterectomy for asymptomatic carotid artery stenosis. JAMA 1995;273(18):1421–8.

[6] Mead GE, Murray H, Farrell A, et al. Pilot study of carotid surgery for acute stroke. Br J Surg 1997;84(7):990–2.

[7] Sacco RL, Kargman DE, Gu Q, et al. Race-ethnicity and determinants of intracranial atherosclerotic cerebral infarction. Stroke 1995;26:14–20.

[8] Moody DM, Bell MA, Challa VR. Features of the cerebral vascular pattern that predict vulnerability to perfusion or oxygen deficiency: an anatomic study. AJNR Am J Neuroradiol 1990;11: 431–9.

[9] Jones TH, Morawetz RB, Crowell RM, et al. Thresholds of focal cerebral ischemia in awake monkeys. J Neurosurg 1981;54(6):773–82.

[10] Tekkok SB, Ye Z, Ransom BR. Excitotoxic mechanisms of ischemic injury in myelinated white matter. J Cereb Blood Flow Metab 2007, in press.

[11] Marchal G, Serrati C, Rioux P, et al. PET imaging of cerebral perfusion and oxygen consumption in acute ischemic stroke: relation to outcome. Lancet 1993;341:925–7.

[12] Heiss W-D, Graf R, Weinhard K, et al. Dynamic penumbra demonstrated by sequential multitracer PET after middle cerebral artery occlusion in cats. J Cereb Blood Flow Metab 1994;14: 892–902.

[13] NINDS rt-PA Stroke Group. Tissue plasminogen activator for acute ischemic stroke. N Engl J Med 1995;333:1581–7.

[14] Derdeyn CP, Grubb RL Jr, Powers WJ. Cerebral hemodynamic impairment: methods of measurement and association with stroke risk. Neurology 1999;53(2):251–9.

[15] Derdeyn CP, Videen TO, Yundt KD, et al. Variability of cerebral blood volume and oxygen extraction: stages of cerebral haemodynamic impairment revisited. Brain 2002;125(Pt 3): 595–607.

[16] Kontos HA, Wei EP, Navari RM, et al. Responses of cerebral arteries and arterioles to acute hypotension and hypertension. Am J Physiol 1978; 243:H371–83.

[17] Kontos HA, Wei EP, Raper AJ, et al. Role of tissue hypoxia in local regulation of cerebral microcirculation. Am J Physiol 1978;234:H582–91.

[18] Rapela CE, Green HD. Autoregulation of canine cerebral blood flow. Circ Res 1964;15:I205–11.

[19] Schumann P, Touzani O, Young AR, et al. Evaluation of the ratio of cerebral blood flow to cerebral blood volume as an index of local cerebral perfusion pressure. Brain 1998;121:1369–79.

[20] Lennox WG, Gibbs FA, Gibbs EL. Relationship of unconsciousness to cerebral blood flow and to

anoxemia. Archives of Neurology and Psychiatry 1935;34:1001–13.

[21] Kety SS, King BD, Horvath SM, et al. The effects of an acute reduction in blood pressure by means of differential spinal sympathetic block on the cerebral circulation of hypertensive patients. J Clin Invest 1950;29:402–7.

[22] Mintun MA, Raichle ME, Martin WRW, et al. Brain oxygen utilization measured with O-15 radiotracers and positron emission tomography. J Nucl Med 1984;25:177–87.

[23] Mintun MA, Lundstrom BN, Snyder AZ, et al. Blood flow and oxygen delivery to human brain during functional activity: theoretical modeling and experimental data. Proc Natl Acad Sci U S A 2001;98(12):6859–64.

[24] Derdeyn CP, Shaibani A, Moran CJ, et al. Lack of correlation between pattern of collateralization and misery perfusion in patients with carotid occlusion. Stroke 1999;30(5):1025–32.

[25] Levine RL, Lagreye HL, Dobkin JA, et al. Cerebral vasocapacitance and TIAs. Neurology 1989;39: 25–9.

[26] Beal MF, Williams RS, Richardson EP, et al. Cholesterol embolism as a cause of transient ischemic attacks and cerebral infarction. Neurology 1981;31(7):860–5.

[27] del Zoppo GJ, Poeck K, Pessin MS, et al. Recombinant tissue plasminogen activator in acute thrombotic and embolic stroke. Ann Neurol 1992;32(1):78–86.

[28] Zanette EM, Fieschi C, Bozzao L, et al. Comparison of cerebral angiography and transcranial Doppler sonography in acute stroke. Stroke 1989;20:899–903.

[29] Horowitz SH, Zito JL, Donnarumma R, et al. Computed tomographic—angiographic findings within the first five hours of cerebral infarction. Stroke 1991;22:1245–53.

[30] Bozzao L, Fantozzi LM, Bastianello S, et al. Ischaemic supratentorial stroke: angiographic findings in patients examined in the very early phase. J Neurol 1989;236:340–2.

[31] Wessels T, Rottger C, Jauss M, et al. Identification of embolic stroke patterns by diffusion-weighted MRI in clinically defined lacunar stroke syndromes. Stroke 2005;36(4):757–61.

[32] Kang DW, Chu K, Ko SB, et al. Lesion patterns and mechanism of ischemia in internal carotid artery disease: a diffusion-weighted imaging study. Arch Neurol 2002;59(10):1577–82.

[33] Molloy J, Markus HS. Asymptomatic embolization predicts stroke and TIA risk in patients with carotid artery stenosis. Stroke 1999;30: 1440–3.

[34] Grubb RL Jr, Derdeyn CP, Fritsch SM, et al. Importance of hemodynamic factors in the prognosis of symptomatic carotid occlusion. JAMA 1998;280(12):1055–60.

[35] Powers WJ. Cerebral hemodynamics in ischemic cerebrovascular disease. Ann Neurol 1991;29:231–40.

[36] Silvestrini M, Troisi E, Matteis M, et al. Transcranial Doppler assessment of cerebrovascular reactivity in symptomatic and asymptomatic severe carotid stenosis. Stroke 1996;27:1970–3.

[37] Yamauchi H, Fukuyama H, Nagahama Y, et al. Significance of increased oxygen extraction fraction in five-year prognosis of major cerebral arterial occlusive disease. J Nucl Med 1999;40: 1992–8.

[38] Vernieri F, Pasqualetti P, Passarelli F, et al. Outcome of carotid artery occlusion is predicted by cerebrovascular reactivity. Stroke 1999;30: 593–8.

[39] Waterston JA, Brown MM, Butler P, et al. Small deep cerebral infarcts associated with occlusive internal carotid artery disease. A hemodynamic phenomenon? Arch Neurol 1990;47:953–7.

[40] Derdeyn CP, Khosla A, Videen TO, et al. Severe hemodynamic impairment and border zone–region infarction. Radiology 2001;220(1): 195–201.

[41] Weiller C, Ringelstein EB, Reiche W, et al. Clinical and hemodynamic aspects of low-flow infarcts. Stroke 1991;22:1117–23.

[42] Yamauchi H, Fukuyama H, Yamaguchi S, et al. High-intensity area in the deep white matter indicating hemodynamic compromise in internal carotid artery occlusive disorders. Arch Neurol 1991;48:1067–71.

[43] Krapf H, Widder B, Skalej M. Small rosary-like infarctions in the centrum semiovale suggest hemodynamic failure. AJNR Am J Neuroradiol 1998;19:1479–84.

[44] Isaka Y, Nagano K, Narita M, et al. High signal intensity on T2-weighted magnetic resonance imaging and cerebral hemodynamic reserve in carotid occlusive disease. Stroke 1997;28:354–7.

[45] Torvik A, Skellerud K. Watershed infarcts in the brain caused by microemboli. Clin Neuropathol 1982;1:99–105.

[46] Pollanen MS, Deck JH. Directed embolization is an alternate cause of cerebral watershed infarction. Arch Pathol Lab Med 1989;113(10): 1139–41.

[47] Adams JH, Brierley JB, Connor RCJ, et al. The effects of systemic hypotension upon the human brain: clinical and neuropathologic observations in 11 cases. Brain 1966;89:235–68.

[48] Derdeyn CP, Simmons NR, Videen TO, et al. Absence of selective deep white matter ischemia in chronic carotid disease: a positron emission tomographic study of regional oxygen extraction. AJNR Am J Neuroradiol 2000;21(4):631–8.

[49] Mull M, Schwarz M, Thron A. Cerebral hemispheric low-flow infarcts in arterial occlusive disease. Lesion patterns and angiomorphological conditions. Stroke 1997;28:118–23.

[50] Derdeyn CP, Yundt KD, Videen TO, et al. Increased oxygen extraction fraction is associated with prior ischemic events in patients with carotid occlusion. Stroke 1998;29(4):754–8.

[51] Omae T, Mayzel-Oreg O, Li F, et al. Inapparent hemodynamic insufficiency exacerbates ischemic damage in a rat microembolic stroke model. Stroke 2000;31:2494–9.

[52] De Ley G, Nshimyumuremyi JB, Leusen J. Hemispheric blood flow in the rat after unilateral carotid common carotid occlusion: evaluation with time. Stroke 1985;16:69–73.

[53] Coyle P, Panzenbeck MJ. Collateral development after carotid artery occlusion in Fischer 344 rats. Stroke 1990;21:316–21.

[54] Endres M, Laufs U, Huang Z, et al. Stroke protection by 3-hydroxy-3-methylglutary (HMG)-CoA reductase inhibitors mediated by endothelial

nitric oxide synthase. Proc Natl Acad Sci U S A 1998;95:8880–5.

[55] Pullicino P, Mifsud V, Wong E, et al. Hypoperfusion-related cerebral ischemia and cardiac left ventricular systolic dysfunction. J Stroke Cerebrovasc Dis 2001;10(4):178–82.

[56] Caplan LR, Hennerici M. Impaired clearance of emboli (washout) is an important link between hypoperfusion, embolism, and ischemic stroke. Arch Neurol 1998;55(11):1475–82.

[57] Silvestrini M, Vernieri F, Pasqualetti P, et al. Impaired cerebral vasoreactivity and risk of stroke in patients with asymptomatic carotid artery stenosis. JAMA 2000;283:2122–7.

NEUROIMAGING CLINICS OF NORTH AMERICA

Neuroimag Clin N Am 17 (2007) 313–324

Chronic Ischemia and Neurocognition

Mohamad Chmayssani, MD, Joanne R. Festa, PhD,
Randolph S. Marshall, MD, MS*

- Evidence of impaired cognition due to carotid artery disease
- Mechanisms
  Hypoperfusion
  Embolization
- *Lacunar disease*
- Chronic ischemia and neuronal impairment
- Summary
- References

Chronic ischemia is a progressive condition caused by cerebral hypoperfusion that ultimately leads to neuronal death. The impact of hypoperfusion on cerebral function has been described in various clinical settings. Acutely systemic hypoperfusion can cause dizziness, visual disturbance, impaired cognition, and loss of consciousness, but, in that setting, cerebral hypoperfusion is easily reversible by laying the patient horizontally and restoring an adequate level of blood pressure. In subacute and chronic settings, cognitive brain functions are affected when the brain is subject to a sustained reduction of blood flow, as may occur in carotid artery disease. The degree, volume, and the duration of hypoperfusion are all variables that influence the brain's response to chronic ischemia. Additional factors, such as pre-existing white-matter disease, cardiac status, thromboembolism, and medical comorbidities, all may contribute to determining whether carotid artery disease produces cognitive impairment. In this article, the authors review the clinical evidence for cognitive dysfunction in carotid artery disease and consider the evidence for chronic ischemia as an underlying pathophysiologic mechanism for cognitive impairment.

Evidence of impaired cognition due to carotid artery disease

Cognitive impairment has been reported in a wide spectrum of clinical studies in patients who have carotid disease, most frequently in global terms rather than as a specific, neurocognitive profile. Fischer [1,2] was the first to postulate an association between cerebral hypoperfusion and dementia, based on a necropsy study of a demented patient who had bilateral carotid occlusion. A few years later, Carey and colleagues [3] reported dementia in four patients who had bilateral carotid occlusion and two patients who had unilateral carotid artery occlusion. Cognitive dysfunction that results from large cortical infarction in territories supplied by carotid arteries is easy to understand; the causative relationship between carotid disease and cognitive functions is less clear when major stroke does not occur.

This article was supported by NIH grant R01 NS048212-01A1 and the Richard and Jenny Levine Research Fund.
Department of Neurology, Division of Stroke and Critical Care, Columbia University Medical Center, 710 West 168th Street, New York, NY 10032, USA
* Corresponding author.
E-mail address: rsm2@columbia.edu (R.S. Marshall).

doi:10.1016/j.nic.2007.03.002

Bakker and colleagues [4] performed an extensive review of literature evaluating cognitive dysfunction in patients with occlusive carotid disease. The lack of recovery from injury due to infarction was not the only means of producing cognitive dysfunction with carotid disease [4]; cognitive impairment was documented among patients who had transient ischemic attack [5–10] and patients with no focal neurologic deficits [7,11,12]. Bakker and colleagues [13] conducted their own study of 39 patients with carotid occlusion who had ipsilateral cerebral or retinal transient ischemic attacks but no stroke on MR imaging. The investigators illustrated significant cognitive impairment in these patients, even in those who had only retinal symptoms and negative MR imaging. Among studies that documented cognitive dysfunction without stroke, two noted a generalized impairment [5,12], three demonstrated focal deficits (memory [7,8], learning [8], psychomotor [7], and problem solving [8,11]), and two did not specify the nature of cognitive deficits [6,10]. Several studies have also demonstrated no relationship between carotid stenosis and cognitive dysfunction [14–17].

Although associations between carotid stenosis and cognitive impairment have been reported widely, the question of cause and effect has been controversial. Mathiesen and colleagues [18] assessed neuropsychologic performance in 189 asymptomatic carotid stenosis patients and found that scores were significantly lower in tests of attention, memory, and psychomotor and motor functioning, compared with 202 patients who had no carotid disease. Cortical infarcts were distributed equally between patients and controls, however, from which they concluded that cognitive dysfunction was unlikely to be caused by emboli from the carotid arteries. Furthermore, because the study patients had relatively low-grade stenosis, hemodynamic insufficiency was also deemed an unlikely causative mechanism. Because lacunar infarcts were more prevalent in the stenosis group, the investigators concluded that carotid stenosis was no more than a marker for underlying generalized atherosclerosis, which was the direct culprit for cognitive dysfunction.

The notion that carotid atherosclerosis is simply a marker for underlying vascular disease was supported also by correlations between neuropsychologic decline and common carotid artery intima-media thickness [19–23] because intima-media thickness reflects the burden of atherosclerosis without requiring stenosis of the internal carotid artery. Hofman and colleagues [21], for example, reported that the presence of carotid plaque and intima-media thickness was associated positively with Alzheimer's disease and vascular dementia.

On the other side of the argument, Johnston and colleagues [24] reasoned that if carotid stenosis was simply a marker of vascular disease, then a similar pattern of cognitive dysfunction should be observed with either left-sided or right-sided carotid disease when using a test such as the Modified Mini-Mental Status Exam, which assesses mainly left hemisphere function. They prospectively followed for 5 years, 4006 patients from the Cardiovascular Health Study, in which high-grade stenosis was present in the left internal carotid artery in 28 participants and the right internal carotid artery in 20 participants. They found that, after adjusting for other vascular risk factors, left-sided stenosis (>75%) was disproportionately associated with cognitive impairment on the Modified Mini-Mental Status Exam, suggesting that carotid stenosis was, in fact, a causative variable. In this study, intima-media thickness was not found to be associated independently with cognitive impairment after adjustment of other risk factors.

Mechanisms

Hypoperfusion

The refinement of new imaging techniques that measure cerebral hemodynamics directly has advanced our understanding of the relationship between hypoperfusion in carotid diseases and cognitive impairment. Tatemichi and colleagues [25] documented the case of a 55-year-old man with bilateral internal carotid and unilateral vertebral artery occlusions presenting with a subacute onset of severe behavioral and cognitive changes. Quantitative cerebral blood flow (CBF) and positron emission tomography (PET) studies showed a 40% to 50% reduction in blood flow and metabolism. Following extracranial/intracranial (EC/IC) bypass, the patient demonstrated an appreciable neuropsychologic improvement that was accompanied by significant increases in CBF and metabolism. Another study integrating data about cognitive performance, CBF, and metabolism showed that 25 patients who had unilateral carotid occlusion and poor neuropsychologic performance had significantly reduced regional CBF (rCBF), regional cerebrovascular reactivity, and regional cerebral metabolic rate for oxygen (rCMRO$_2$) [26]. Another PET study showed that 12 patients who had significant cognitive dysfunction had a wide spread of metabolic derangement [27]. Finally, using single photon emission computed tomography (SPECT), Tsuda and colleagues [28] documented the case of a patient diagnosed with total occlusion left internal carotid artery siphon presenting with a generalized, cognitive impairment in the ipsilateral hemisphere. His cognitive status was coupled to an extensive hypoperfusion area in the left anterior parietal and parietotemporal cortex.

Additional evidence for the effects of chronic cerebral hypoperfusion on cognitive function comes from the cardiac literature. End-stage heart failure may produce a state of global ischemia of the brain resembling the state resulting from hypoperfusion due to carotid disease. Recent studies have found that as many as 35% to 50% of patients who have heart failure have a cognitive dysfunction [28–31]. The pathophysiology of cognitive impairment in end-stage heart failure has been attributed to hypoperfusion and microembolism [32]. The most widely accepted view is that decreased cardiac pumping efficiency directly influences cerebral perfusion [30]. In human subjects, global CBF reductions have been reported in heart failure patients using functional imaging studies with SPECT [33–36].

In a pioneering study, Gruhn and colleagues [36] demonstrated that CBF was reduced by approximately 31% in 12 patients (36 ± 1 mL/min per 100 g), when compared with 12 healthy subjects (52 ± 5 mL/min per 100 g) ($P < .05$). Among the studied subjects, five patients underwent heart transplantation that resulted in a significant increase in CBF, from 35 ± 3 to 50 ± 3 mL/min per 100 g within the first month postoperation ($P < .05$). Another study showed that cardiac recipients had an increase in cardiac output that resulted in a concomitant increase in middle cerebral artery (MCA)-mean flow velocity [36]. Although neither study included neuropsychologic testing of patients, the significant 31% increase in CBF may offer a physiologic explanation for clinical reports of neuropsychologic improvement following cardiac transplantation [37–39].

Data from studies prospectively evaluating the cognitive status of patients undergoing cardiac transplants contain some evidence for cognitive change. One report failed to demonstrate significant cognitive improvement in 54 patients who were assessed preoperatively, 20 of whom completed postoperative testing [40]. On the other hand, three prospective reports evaluating cognition among cardiac recipients showed improvement in cognitive performance of various functions [37–39]. The enhanced cortical perfusion following transplant is felt to be the cause of improvement in attention span and reduction in depression and anxiety [37,41,42].

Pacemaker implantation is another approach by which cognition can be improved potentially in patients who have heart dysfunction [43,44]. Pacemakers improve heart rate, resulting in increased CBF levels [43]. Illustratively, Koide and colleagues [43] reported an improvement in CBF and verbal intelligence following pacemaker implantation in 14 bradycardiac patients.

Carotid artery stenting/carotid endarterectomy

In a manner analogous to the cognitive improvement following CBF increases with treatment of heart dysfunction, studies that demonstrate cognitive improvement following revascularization support the hypoperfusion hypothesis.

Many studies have evaluated the effect of carotid endarterectomy (CE) on cognitive functioning. Results have been variable, ranging from benefit, to decrease, to no change. In reviews by Irvine and colleagues [45] and Lunn and colleagues [46] in the late 1990s, 16 of 28 studies (57%) reported cognitive improvement following CE, whereas deterioration was reported in 1 report (4%) and no change in 11 reports (39%).

Subsequent studies of CE have shown some support for the hypoperfusion hypothesis. Among those demonstrating cognitive benefit [47–50], the positive impact on cognition was attributed to a significant increase in CBF [49] or to a reduced preoperative cerebral perfusion reserve [50,51]. However, other studies have found no restorative effect on cognition [51–53]. A recent study showed that after 44 months of postoperative follow-up, cognitive dysfunction occurred in almost one half of patients who underwent CE, and the decline was more prominent in symptomatic patients who had left internal carotid artery disease than in asymptomatic patients who had left internal carotid artery disease or in patients who had right internal carotid artery disease, either symptomatic or asymptomatic [54].

Some studies investigated side-specific cognitive effects, based on the premise that restoration of hemodynamic physiologic conditions would be more beneficial to the cognitive functions of the cerebral hemisphere ipsilateral to the operated side. This hypothesis stems from pre- and postoperative MR imaging studies, in which ipsilateral white-matter changes were reported to be reversible to a certain extent by endarterectomy [55]. However, no solid conclusion was reached in these studies regarding side-related benefits of CE on cognition [50,51].

Controversy prevails and, consequently, final conclusions regarding the impact of CE on cognition cannot be reached. The wide spectrum in results, ranging from a decline, to no effect, to a benefit, has been explained by periprocedural complications [56–58] and differences in methodologic factors, such as battery of neuropsychologic testing, sample size and use of control population, severity of carotid stenosis, associated comorbidities, and time to postoperative follow-up [45,46,57].

Because of the neurologic variability, no consistent cognitive profile exists for patients who have carotid disease.

Carotid artery stenting came into routine clinical practice only in the last decade; for this reason, knowledge about the effect of carotid artery stenting on cognition is limited, but it is presumed to follow the same principle as CE. Lehrner and colleagues [59] studied the cognitive outcome of 20 patients, 9 symptomatic with transient ischemic attack and 11 asymptomatic, 6 months after unilateral carotid stenting. Most patients had no significant change in cognitive functioning. On the other hand, 10 patients assessed 48 hours post-op showed an improvement of cognitive status following carotid artery stenting [60]. Another study compared cognitive outcome in 20 patients undergoing carotid angioplasty without stenting with 26 patients undergoing CE. At 6 weeks follow-up, five patients in each group had a comparable decline in cognition [61]. As with CE studies, it was shown that improvement in perfusion parameters following stent deployment, carotid or vertebrobasilar, was a significant predictor of cognitive improvement [62].

Extracranial/intracranial bypass

EC/IC bypass surgery was used commonly during the 1970s and early 1980s to treat patients who had total occlusion of carotid arteries and were not candidates for carotid endarterectomy. The fact that intellectual decline has been linked to chronic ischemia set the ground for investigators to address the efficacy of EC/IC bypass in restoring cognitive functions. The concept of blood flow restitution is the pillar on which EC/IC bypass surgery is based. However, the effectiveness of EC/IC bypass was reported initially only in case studies. For instance, Nielsen and colleagues [63] found that among 33 patients undergoing EC/IC bypass, 23 had preoperative impairment of cognition that improved 3 months after surgery. A case series of 38 patients being referred for EC/IC bypass showed an improvement in scores of neuropsychologic tests of processing speed and memory [64]. Binder and colleagues [65] compared the cognition of 12 patients undergoing EC/IC bypass with 7 patients who had internal carotid artery occlusion treated medically. Limited to only 2 months of follow-up, no significant difference was detected. Of note, the previous studies [63–65] had no control subjects, nor any hemodynamic data.

Reports from that era that assessed CBF changes following EC/IC bypass are also conflicting. Younkin and colleagues [9] conducted a study without controls and evaluated CBF with a ^{133}Xe inhalation technique in a series of 44 patients undergoing EC/IC bypass. Neuropsychologic performance increased at 3 months and further improvement was detected at 9 months; however, the clinical improvement was not associated with similar changes in CBF values. A maximum increase in CBF at 3 months was noted, followed by a decrease to preoperative baseline levels by 9 months. Yonekura and colleagues [66] found no changes in CBF measures at 6 months and decreased measures at 2 years, but Halsey and colleagues [67] reported a significant increase in CBF at 6 months.

The initial evidence regarding the impact of EC/IC bypass on hemodynamics and cognitive functions is contentious. However, several studies did correlate cognitive postoperative changes with cerebral hemodynamics. Using SPECT, Tsuda and colleagues [28] documented a case where the recovery in blood flow and metabolic rate following EC/IC bypass was translated into improvement in both neurologic and cognitive functions. During a period of 3 to 9 months postoperatively, rCBF was normalized, whereas cognitive improvement was witnessed in the first 2 postoperative months and maintained over a 3-year follow-up. In a more recent investigation, Sasoh and colleagues [26] studied 25 patients who had chronic cerebral ischemia due to internal carotid occlusion, who underwent pre- and postoperative measurement of CBF and metabolism using PET. They demonstrated that elevated regional oxygen extraction rate and reduced cerebral metabolic rate for oxygen ($CMRO_2$) were associated strongly with cognitive impairment. Postoperatively, the hemodynamic factors increased significantly, accompanied by significant improvement in verbal IQ, performance, and full-scale IQ scores. Their hemodynamic findings were consistent with previous studies that demonstrated restitution of rCBF, oxygen extraction rate and $CMRO_2$ following EC/IC bypass [68–71]. This effect of EC/IC bypass on cognition in patients who had stage II hemodynamic failure was the basis for initiating the currently active Randomized Evaluation of Carotid Occlusion and Neurocognition, in which patients' cognitive function over 2 years will be compared in an National Institutes of Health–sponsored, prospective, randomized clinical trial. Patients will receive either EC/IC bypass or best medical therapy alone as part of the Carotid Occlusion Surgery Study.

Embolization

In addition to hypoperfusion, brain damage secondary to carotid disease may be produced by episodic embolization of platelet, thrombotic, or cholesterol material with microinfarction of cerebral tissue [72]. Using random transcranial Doppler monitoring, spontaneous microemboli can be detected in 21% to 60% of patients who have documented carotid disease [73–77].

Emboli reaching one hemisphere or retina commonly stem from the ipsilateral carotid, and, in particular, from the distal or proximal stump, or from atherosclerotic plaques in the common carotid artery [78–80]. Transhemispheric emboli (ie, microemboli) causing ischemic events in the contralateral hemisphere also may occur [81]. Ischemic events due to microemboli occurring in the brain hemisphere ipsilateral to the occluded internal carotid artery are reduced after clipping of the proximal stump [79], following endarterectomy in contralateral internal carotid artery stenosis [81], or after use of antithrombotic agents [79].

Whether microembolism from carotid disease is clinically significant remains an open question. Droste and colleagues [76] detected up to 142 embolic signals per hour in patients who had carotid stenosis and a recent transient ischemic attack; however, symptoms developing as a result of these embolic showers occur at a surprisingly low rate [56,82–84], perhaps because of collateral washout. Older age, hypertension, diabetes, or small-vessel disease appear to increase the susceptibility of the brain to injury from microemboli [85]. Acute ischemic events also have a size threshold [85,86], larger emboli being more likely to cause symptoms [84]. Furthermore, transient symptoms might go unnoticed in patients experiencing microembolization during sleep [87].

Even if microembolism does not induce immediate consequences, delayed sequelae are possible. Embolic fragments may trigger an inflammatory process that, in time, leads to cellular infiltration and fibrosis [88,89]. This phenomenon could account for late deterioration in cognitive functions, as it does in patients following coronary artery bypass [90,91].

Lacunar disease

A growing literature suggests that white-matter lesions are involved in the pathogenesis of cognitive impairment [92–104], more so in the periventricular than subcortical regions [50,95,105,106], periventricular lesions showing a strong relationship with memory, psychomotor, and global cognitive dysfunctions [95]. Severe carotid disease of 70% stenosis is associated with deep white-matter lesions and lacunar infarction [107–109].

One study showed that carotid artery narrowing of more than 50% is an independent predictor of lacunar infarction [109], which, in turn, is associated significantly with attention deficits and frontal lobe dysfunction. The clinical significance of asymptomatic cerebral microinfarction was recognized in the Rotterdam Scan Study, which showed

that the incidence of silent infarcts detected by MR imaging among healthy elderly patients doubles the risk of developing cognitive decline on follow-up [110]. Suffering additional silent infarcts appears to promote further cognitive deterioration [111]. These findings were reproduced in two large studies, the Atherosclerosis Risk in Communities Study [112] and the Cardiovascular Health Study [113]. Silent infarcts of both white matter [114–116] and cortical gray matter [117] also have been correlated with poor cognition [110].

From the clinical data presented, it appears that cognitive impairment in carotid disease may result from small-vessel disease, microembolism, or chronic hypoperfusion (**Fig. 1**). It is the last that has been most difficult to characterize physiologically. What follows is a review of the experimental literature that supports the existence of chronic ischemia in the brain.

Chronic ischemia and neuronal impairment

If hypoperfusion is the primary model for the link between carotid disease and cognitive impairment, one must provide evidence that

Chronic ischemia exists and results in neuronal dysfunction.

Chronic ischemia and neuronal dysfunction are reversible.

Chronic ischemia and reversibility correlate with functional behavioral measures.

Animal studies can provide a pure model of chronic cerebral hypoperfusion. Ohta and colleagues [118] investigated the effect of chronic cerebral ischemia on learning behaviors in rats. They compared a novel rat cerebral hypoperfusion model of bilateral internal carotid artery ligation (BICL) with a previously established model of bilateral common carotid artery ligation (BCCL).

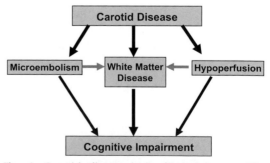

Fig. 1. Carotid disease is implicated in cognitive impairment through three direct mechanisms: (1) microembolism, (2) white-matter disease, and (3) hypoperfusion. Microembolism and hypoperfusion further contribute to cognitive impairment by increasing the burden of white-matter disease.

The rats were tested by measuring the escape latencies in the Morris water maze task and eight-arm radial mask. Both groups had a significant reduction in CBF at day 10, although the reduction was less extensive in BICL rats than in BCCL rats. This graded difference in reduction in CBF between the two groups was reflected in a graded behavioral performance. Both groups of rats demonstrated poor performance in the eight-arm radial mask task, whereas in the Morris water maze task, the BCCL rats performed more poorly than the BICL rats. Histopathologic analysis showed that the BCCL rats had major rarefaction and gliosis of the white matter and neuronal infarction in the hippocampal CA1 region; on the contrary, BICL rats had no significant brain damage. For this reason, it was inferred that behavioral impairment in the BICL rats was caused by an isolated decrease in CBF without infarction and, therefore, that neuronal loss is not a prerequisite for cognitive dysfunction [118].

Several other rat studies have also demonstrated that hypoperfusion can lead to learning and memory deficits as late as 1 to 6 weeks following carotid occlusion[119–124]. Again, in these studies [119,120], behavioral impairment was evident before hippocampal damage was seen, suggesting further that hypoperfusion, without the presence of cellular damage, can produce learning and memory deficits. Recently, a multistage carotid occlusion technique was evaluated as a hypoperfusion model in rats, and this study showed similar effects. Within 4 weeks, persistent cognitive impairment was established, and only 49 days later, hippocampal neuronal loss was seen [125].

Rat models of chronic ischemia have shown that neurons are capable of existing in a suspended metabolic state when either no energy substrates [126] or diminished energy substrates [127,128] are available. This reduced metabolic state was characterized more precisely by showing that the ischemic thresholds for neuronal electric failure and for neuronal metabolic failure resulting in neuronal death are distinct [129]. At the threshold of electrical failure [130,131] (0.1 mL/min per 100 g), ion homeostasis is still maintained, suggesting that normal cellular functions can be restored potentially, because neurons remain intact. The integrity of neurons is reflected by a minimal, if any, increase in extracellular potassium concentration, which is indicative of ion pump failure. A further reduction in blood flow below the flow threshold for energy failure results in ATP depletion, a massive increase in extracellular potassium, and subsequent neuronal death [129]. At the threshold of electrical failure, neuronal energy stores are preserved at nearly normal levels.

Odano and colleagues [132] also demonstrated that a prolonged hypometabolic state can exist in viable cells. They conducted a histopathologic study in gerbils with chronic infarction due to middle cerebral artery (MCA) occlusion, using a SPECT dual tracer technique of glucose metabolism and iomazenil, SPECT ligand for central benzodiazepine receptors useful as an indicator of integrity of cortical neurons. Based on histopathologic examinations, cells that were damaged severely had low [^{14}C]-2-DG and low iomazenil bindings, whereas cells with only mild neuronal degenerations had low uptake of [^{14}C]-2-DG but almost normal levels of iomazenil uptake. Those findings strongly suggest that neurons can exist at a hypofunctional but viable state for a prolonged period of time in the setting of decreased CBF and metabolism.

If cells can remain viable when subjected to prolonged ischemia, the question that follows is whether it is possible for hypofunctional cells to resume normal metabolic rates if physiologic conditions are restored. The clinical correlate would be the improvement in cognitive performance described in studies following carotid revascularization.

de la Torre and colleagues [133] subjected middle-aged rats to bilateral common carotid artery and left subclavian artery occlusion, which produce chronic cerebrovascular insufficiency resulting in selective CA1 damage in the hippocampus [127,134]. Three groups of rats had their CBF restored after 1, 2, or 3 weeks by undergoing deocclusion of the vessels. These rats were assessed behaviorally and histopathologically at 9 weeks and were compared with another group of rats that did not undergo deocclusion of the vessels. The investigators found that the permanent occlusion and the 3-week occlusion group failed to regain their memory deficit and had a high degree of reactive astrocytic hypertrophy. In contrast, rats that underwent deocclusion at 1 or 2 weeks had less neuronal damage and less reactive astrocytic hypertrophy, compared with those whose clips stayed on the full 3 weeks. At 9 weeks, the early deocclusion groups performed well on the spatial memory tasks. Local cerebral blood flow (LCBF) was measured at the beginning of the experiment and 9 weeks later in all rat groups. At the end of the 9-week experimental period, all three deoccluded rat groups had LCBF levels similar to intact control, whereas rats subjected to permanent ischemia had a significant decrease in LCBF in the frontoparietal cortex. The investigators concluded that neuronal cells may exist in a reversible state of chronic ischemia for a prolonged amount of time.

Although animal model evidence appears fairly convincing for the pathophysiologic entity of chronic, reversible ischemia, four hemodynamic parameters are likely to influence the brain's response to the hypoperfusion of carotid artery

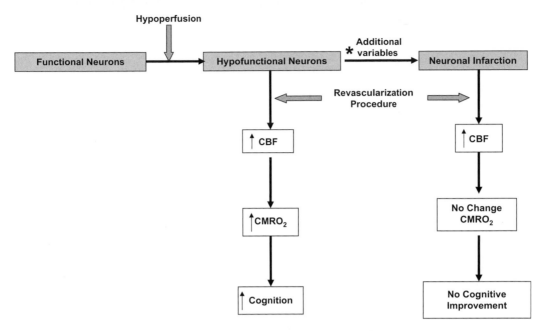

* Microembolism, White matter dz, prolonged hypoperfusion, Increased severity of hypoperfusion, Increased volume of ischemia

Fig. 2. Proposed natural history of neurons subjected to chronic ischemia. Hypoperfusion shifts cells into a hypo-functional, but viable, state. If a revascularization procedure is done at that point, a resultant increase in CBF leads to a concomitant increase in neuronal metabolism, and this manifests in improved cognitive performance. On the other hand, if the hypoperfusion state is prolonged, increased in severity or volume, or coexists with either microemboli or white-matter disease, infarction occurs and revascularization will result in a CBF restoration that does produce increased neuronal metabolism or consequent cognitive improvement.

disease in humans: degree of hypoperfusion, duration of hypoperfusion, rapidity of onset of hypoperfusion, and volume of hypoperfusion.

Using a xenon-CBF washout technique to measure hemispheral blood flow quantitatively, Marshall and colleagues [135] studied delineated CBF thresholds for cognition experimentally in the setting of carotid artery balloon test occlusions. Although this experiment measured cognitive change in an acute setting, it provides useful quantitative data that may be applicable in the chronic setting. Using a sustained attention task in which patients were required to press a mouse button continuously every 10 to 13 seconds, the deterioration of sustained attention performance was found to correlate with the abruptness and degree of reduction in CBF. One group maintained normal sustained attention performance throughout the carotid occlusion test. This group had a mean CBF of 47 mL/min per 100g. A second group of patients with a lower CBF measuring 37 mL/min per 100g had an initial transient drop in attention that resolved after a few minutes, despite persistent carotid test occlusion. A third group of patients also experienced an initial drop in attention; however, they did not return to baseline sustained attention

performance until the balloon was deflated at the end of the test. This group had the lowest CBF values, averaging 27 mL/min per 100g. This experiment illustrates that both time course and severity of blood flow reduction determine the impact of hypoperfusion on cognitive function. In chronic ischemia settings, time appears to work against neuronal adaptation to low-flow states, leading to a stage of irreversibility, as exemplified in the study conducted by de la Torre and colleagues [133] and in the animal studies [118–120], which showed behavioral impairment preceding hippocampal neuronal damage as a result of carotid ligation.

The last qualitative parameter of chronic ischemia is the volume of cortex that is subject to chronic ischemia. A volume effect was illustrated in the study conducted by Ohta and colleagues [118]; BCCL rats with larger hypoperfused territory and lower CBF values had more hippocampal neuronal damage and more behavioral impairment, compared with BICL rats. In humans, volume of hypoperfusion depends directly on the efficiency of collateralization within the circle of Willis and over the cortical convexity [136]. The better the collateralization, the less likely that chronic ischemia will be irreversible.

In summary, ischemia is more likely to be irreversible when neurons are subject to hypoperfusion that is of longer duration, more severe, of larger volume, or more abrupt. In a clinical setting, severity of hypoperfusion can be estimated using blood flow studies such as PET, SPECT, CT perfusion or MR perfusion imaging. Estimations of adequacy of collateral flow (volume of ischemia) can be made with techniques such as transcranial Doppler. However, acuity of onset and duration of hypoperfusion are ascertained less easily. Furthermore, additional co-morbidities, such as prior cerebral infarcts, chronic cardiac or other systemic disease, or primary neuro-degenerative processes, ultimately need to be factored into the equation in trying to predict whether cognitive dysfunction in any given individual is likely to occur. Moreover, additional research is needed to characterize better the cognitive profile of patients who have carotid disease.

Summary

Substantial evidence indicates that chronic ischemia is a progressive, dynamic process that may manifest with cognitive dysfunction as the ischemic conditions persist, with functional deficits becoming evident and additional neuronal infarction prevailing if chronic ischemia is not reversed. By incorporating the pathophysiology of chronic ischemia into the algorithm of the management of carotid artery disease, we may be able to extend the goals of carotid artery revascularization beyond merely preventing stroke to include the prospect of preventing or reversing cognitive decline (Fig. 2).

References

[1] Fisher M. Senile dementia—a new explanation of its causation. Can Med Assoc J 1951;65(1): 1–7.

[2] Fisher M. Occlusion of the carotid arteries: further experiences. AMA Arch Neurol Psychiatry 1954;72(2):187–204.

[3] Carey JB Jr, Wilson ID, Zaki FG, et al. The metabolism of bile acids with special reference to liver injury. Medicine (Baltimore) 1966;45(6): 461–70.

[4] Bakker FC, Klijn CJ, Jennekens-Schinkel A, et al. Cognitive disorders in patients with occlusive disease of the carotid artery: a systematic review of the literature. J Neurol 2000;247(9):669–76.

[5] Hemmingsen R, Mejsholm B, Boysen G, et al. Intellectual function in patients with transient ischaemic attacks (TIA) or minor stroke. Long-term improvement after carotid endarterectomy. Acta Neurol Scand 1982;66(2):145–59.

[6] Baird AD, Adams KM, Shatz MW, et al. Can neuropsychological tests detect the sites of cerebrovascular stenoses and occlusions? Neurosurgery 1984;14(4):416–23.

[7] Hamster W, Diener HC. Neuropsychological changes associated with stenoses or occlusions of the carotid arteries. A comparative psychometric study. Eur Arch Psychiatry Neurol Sci 1984;234(1):69–73.

[8] Nielsen H, Hojer-Pedersen E, Gulliksen G, et al. A neuropsychological study of 12 patients with transient ischemic attacks before and after EC/IC bypass surgery. Acta Neurol Scand 1985; 71(4):317–20.

[9] Younkin D, Hungerbuhler JP, O'Connor M, et al. Superficial temporal-middle cerebral artery anastomosis: effects on vascular, neurologic, and neuropsychological functions. Neurology 1985;35(4):462–9.

[10] Hemmingsen R, Mejsholm B, Vorstrup S, et al. Carotid surgery, cognitive function, and cerebral blood flow in patients with transient ischemic attacks. Ann Neurol 1986;20(1):13–9.

[11] Naugle RI, Bridgers SL, Delaney RC. Neuropsychological signs of asymptomatic carotid stenosis [brief report]. Arch Clin Neuropsychol 1986;1:25–30.

[12] Benke T, Neussl D, Aichner F. Neuropsychological deficits in asymptomatic carotid artery stenosis. Acta Neurol Scand 1991;83(6):378–81.

[13] Bakker FC, Klijn CJ, Jennekens-Schinkel A, et al. Cognitive impairment in patients with carotid artery occlusion and ipsilateral transient ischemic attacks. J Neurol 2003;250(11):1340–7.

[14] Kelly MP, Garron DC, Javid H. Carotid artery disease, carotid endarterectomy, and behavior. Arch Neurol 1980;37(12):743–8.

[15] Boeke S. The effect of carotid endarterectomy on mental functioning. Clin Neurol Neurosurg 1981;83(4):209–17.

[16] van den Burg W, Saan RJ, Van Zomeren AH, et al. Carotid endarterectomy: does it improve cognitive or motor functioning? Psychol Med 1985;15(2):341–6.

[17] Iddon JL, Sahakian BJ, Kirkpatrick PJ. Uncomplicated carotid endarterectomy is not associated with neuropsychological impairment. Pharmacol Biochem Behav 1997;56(4):781–7.

[18] Mathiesen EB, Waterloo K, Joakimsen O, et al. Reduced neuropsychological test performance in asymptomatic carotid stenosis: the Tromso Study. Neurology 2004;62(5):695–701.

[19] Breteler MM, Claus JJ, Grobbee DE, et al. Cardiovascular disease and distribution of cognitive function in elderly people: the Rotterdam Study. BMJ 1994;308(6944):1604–8.

[20] Auperin A, Berr C, Bonithon-Kopp C, et al. Ultrasonographic assessment of carotid wall characteristics and cognitive functions in a community sample of 59- to 71-year-olds. The EVA Study Group. Stroke 1996;27(8):1290–5.

[21] Hofman A, Ott A, Breteler MM, et al. Atherosclerosis, apolipoprotein E, and prevalence of dementia and Alzheimer's disease in the

Rotterdam Study. Lancet 1997;349(9046): 151–4.

[22] Cerhan JR, Folsom AR, Mortimer JA, et al. Correlates of cognitive function in middle-aged adults. Atherosclerosis Risk in Communities (ARIC) Study Investigators. Gerontology 1998; 44(2):95–105.

[23] Kuller LH, Shemanski L, Manolio T, et al. Relationship between ApoE, MRI findings, and cognitive function in the Cardiovascular Health Study. Stroke 1998;29(2):388–98.

[24] Johnston SC, O'Meara ES, Manolio TA, et al. Cognitive impairment and decline are associated with carotid artery disease in patients without clinically evident cerebrovascular disease. Ann Intern Med 2004;140(4):237–47.

[25] Tatemichi TK, Desmond DW, Prohovnik I, et al. Dementia associated with bilateral carotid occlusions: neuropsychological and haemodynamic course after extracranial to intracranial bypass surgery. J Neurol Neurosurg Psychiatry 1995;58(5):633–6.

[26] Sasoh M, Ogasawara K, Kuroda K, et al. Effects of EC-IC bypass surgery on cognitive impairment in patients with hemodynamic cerebral ischemia. Surg Neurol 2003;59(6):455–60. [discussion: 460–3].

[27] Yamauchi H, Fukuyama H, Nagahama Y, et al. Atrophy of the corpus callosum associated with cognitive impairment and widespread cortical hypometabolism in carotid artery occlusive disease. Arch Neurol 1996;53(11): 1103–9.

[28] Tsuda Y, Yamada K, Hayakawa T, et al. Cortical blood flow and cognition after extracranial-intracranial bypass in a patient with severe carotid occlusive lesions. A three-year follow-up study. Acta Neurochir (Wien) 1994;129(3–4):198–204.

[29] Almeida OP, Flicker L. The mind of a failing heart: a systematic review of the association between congestive heart failure and cognitive functioning. Intern Med J 2001;31(5):290–5.

[30] Zuccala G, Onder G, Pedone C, et al. Hypotension and cognitive impairment: selective association in patients with heart failure. Neurology 2001;57(11):1986–92.

[31] Zuccala G, Pedone C, Cesari M, et al. The effects of cognitive impairment on mortality among hospitalized patients with heart failure. Am J Med 2003;115(2):97–103.

[32] Pullicino PM, Hart J. Cognitive impairment in congestive heart failure?: embolism vs hypoperfusion. Neurology 2001;57(11):1945–6.

[33] Rajagopalan B, Raine AE, Cooper R, et al. Changes in cerebral blood flow in patients with severe congestive cardiac failure before and after captopril treatment. Am J Med 1984; 76(5B):86–90.

[34] Kamishirado H, Inoue T, Fujito T, et al. Effect of enalapril maleate on cerebral blood flow in patients with chronic heart failure. Angiology 1997;48(8):707–13.

[35] Georgiadis D, Sievert M, Cencetti S, et al. Cerebrovascular reactivity is impaired in patients with cardiac failure. Eur Heart J 2000;21(5): 407–13.

[36] Gruhn N, Larsen FS, Boesgaard S, et al. Cerebral blood flow in patients with chronic heart failure before and after heart transplantation. Stroke 2001;32(11):2530–3.

[37] Deshields TL, McDonough EM, Mannen RK, et al. Psychological and cognitive status before and after heart transplantation. Gen Hosp Psychiatry 1996;18(Suppl 6):62S–9S.

[38] Grimm M, Yeganehfar W, Laufer G, et al. Cyclosporine may affect improvement of cognitive brain function after successful cardiac transplantation. Circulation 1996;94(6):1339–45.

[39] Roman DD, Kubo SH, Ormaza S, et al. Memory improvement following cardiac transplantation. J Clin Exp Neuropsychol 1997;19(5): 692–7.

[40] Schall RR, Petrucci RJ, Brozena SC, et al. Cognitive function in patients with symptomatic dilated cardiomyopathy before and after cardiac transplantation. J Am Coll Cardiol 1989; 14(7):1666–72.

[41] Jones BM, Chang VP, Esmore D, et al. Psychological adjustment after cardiac transplantation. Med J Aust 1988;149(3):118–22.

[42] Kugler J, Tenderich G, Stahlhut P, et al. Emotional adjustment and perceived locus of control in heart transplant patients. J Psychosom Res 1994;38(5):403–8.

[43] Koide H, Kobayashi S, Kitani M, et al. Improvement of cerebral blood flow and cognitive function following pacemaker implantation in patients with bradycardia. Gerontology 1994; 40(5):279–85.

[44] Barbe C, Puisieux F, Jansen I, et al. Improvement of cognitive function after pacemaker implantation in very old persons with bradycardia. J Am Geriatr Soc 2002;50(4): 778–80.

[45] Irvine CD, Gardner FV, Davies AH, et al. Cognitive testing in patients undergoing carotid endarterectomy. Eur J Vasc Endovasc Surg 1998; 15(3):195–204.

[46] Lunn S, Crawley F, Harrison MJ, et al. Impact of carotid endarterectomy upon cognitive functioning. A systematic review of the literature. Cerebrovasc Dis 1999;9(2):74–81.

[47] Sinforiani E, Curci R, Fancellu R, et al. Neuropsychological changes after carotid endarterectomy. Funct Neurol 2001;16(4):329–36.

[48] Fearn SJ, Hutchinson S, Riding G, et al. Carotid endarterectomy improves cognitive function in patients with exhausted cerebrovascular reserve. Eur J Vasc Endovasc Surg 2003;26(5):529–36.

[49] Kishikawa K, Kamouchi M, Okada Y, et al. Effects of carotid endarterectomy on cerebral blood flow and neuropsychological test performance in patients with high-grade carotid stenosis. J Neurol Sci 2003;213(1–2):19–24.

[50] Fukunaga S, Okada Y, Inoue T, et al. Neuropsychological changes in patients with carotid stenosis after carotid endarterectomy. Eur Neurol 2006;55(3):145–50.

[51] Brand N, Bossema ER, Ommen Mv M, et al. Left or right carotid endarterectomy in patients with atherosclerotic disease: ipsilateral effects on cognition? Brain Cogn 2004;54(2):117–23.

[52] Bossema ER, Brand N, Moll FL, et al. Does carotid endarterectomy improve cognitive functioning? J Vasc Surg 2005;41(5):775–81 [discussion: 781].

[53] Aleksic M, Huff W, Hoppmann B, et al. Cognitive function remains unchanged after endarterectomy of unilateral internal carotid artery stenosis under local anaesthesia. Eur J Vasc Endovasc Surg 2006;31(6):616–21.

[54] Bo M, Massaia M, Speme S, et al. Risk of cognitive decline in older patients after carotid endarterectomy: an observational study. J Am Geriatr Soc 2006;54(6):932–6.

[55] Soinne L, Helenius J, Saimanen E, et al. Brain diffusion changes in carotid occlusive disease treated with endarterectomy. Neurology 2003;61(8):1061–5.

[56] Heyer EJ, DeLaPaz R, Halazun HJ, et al. Neuropsychological dysfunction in the absence of structural evidence for cerebral ischemia after uncomplicated carotid endarterectomy. Neurosurgery 2006;58(3):474–80 [discussion: 474–80].

[57] Ogasawara K, Yamadate K, Kobayashi M, et al. Postoperative cerebral hyperperfusion associated with impaired cognitive function in patients undergoing carotid endarterectomy. J Neurosurg 2005;102(1):38–44.

[58] Jansen C, Sprengers AM, Moll FL, et al. Prediction of intracerebral haemorrhage after carotid endarterectomy by clinical criteria and intraoperative transcranial Doppler monitoring: results of 233 operations. Eur J Vasc Surg 1994;8(2):220–5.

[59] Lehrner J, Willfort A, Mlekusch I, et al. Neuropsychological outcome 6 months after unilateral carotid stenting. J Clin Exp Neuropsychol 2005;27(7):859–66.

[60] Grunwald IQ, Supprian T, Politi M, et al. Cognitive changes after carotid artery stenting. Neuroradiology 2006;48(5):319–23.

[61] Crawley F, Stygall J, Lunn S, et al. Comparison of microembolism detected by transcranial Doppler and neuropsychological sequelae of carotid surgery and percutaneous transluminal angioplasty. Stroke 2000;31(6):1329–34.

[62] Moftakhar R, Turk AS, Niemann DB, et al. Effects of carotid or vertebrobasilar stent placement on cerebral perfusion and cognition. AJNR Am J Neuroradiol 2005;26(7):1772–80.

[63] Nielsen H, Hojer-Pedersen E, Gulliksen G, et al. Reversible ischemic neurological deficit and minor strokes before and after EC/IC bypass surgery. A neuropsychological study. Acta Neurol Scand 1986;73(6):615–8.

[64] Drinkwater JE, Thompson SK, Lumley JS. Cerebral function before and after extra-intracranial carotid bypass. J Neurol Neurosurg Psychiatry 1984;47(9):1041–3.

[65] Binder LM, Tanabe CT, Waller FT, et al. Behavioral effects of superficial temporal artery to middle cerebral artery bypass surgery: preliminary report. Neurology 1982;32(4):422–4.

[66] Yonekura M, Austin G, Hayward W. Long-term evaluation of cerebral blood flow, transient ischemic attacks, and stroke after STA-MCA anastomosis. Surg Neurol 1982;18(2):123–30.

[67] Halsey JH Jr, Morawetz RB, Blauenstein UW. The hemodynamic effect of STA-MCA bypass. Stroke 1982;13(2):163–7.

[68] Powers WJ, Martin WR, Herscovitch P, et al. Extracranial-intracranial bypass surgery: hemodynamic and metabolic effects. Neurology 1984;34(9):1168–74.

[69] Gibbs JM, Wise RJ, Thomas DJ, et al. Cerebral haemodynamic changes after extracranial-intracranial bypass surgery. J Neurol Neurosurg Psychiatry 1987;50(2):140–50.

[70] Takagi Y, Hashimoto N, Iwama T, et al. Improvement of oxygen metabolic reserve after extracranial-intracranial bypass surgery in patients with severe haemodynamic insufficiency. Acta Neurochir (Wien) 1997;139(1):52–6 [discussion: 56–7].

[71] Kobayashi H, Kitai R, Ido K, et al. Hemodynamic and metabolic changes following cerebral revascularization in patients with cerebral occlusive diseases. Neurol Res 1999;21(2):153–60.

[72] Klijn CJ, Kappelle LJ, Tulleken CA, et al. Symptomatic carotid artery occlusion. A reappraisal of hemodynamic factors. Stroke 1997;28(10):2084–93.

[73] Siebler M, Kleinschmidt A, Sitzer M, et al. Cerebral microembolism in symptomatic and asymptomatic high-grade internal carotid artery stenosis. Neurology 1994;44(4):615–8.

[74] Babikian VL, Wijman CA, Hyde C, et al. Cerebral microembolism and early recurrent cerebral or retinal ischemic events. Stroke 1997;28(7):1314–8.

[75] Del Sette M, Angeli S, Stara I, et al. Microembolic signals with serial transcranial Doppler monitoring in acute focal ischemic deficit. A local phenomenon? Stroke 1997;28(7):1311–3.

[76] Droste DW, Hansberg T, Kemeny V, et al. Oxygen inhalation can differentiate gaseous from nongaseous microemboli detected by transcranial Doppler ultrasound. Stroke 1997;28(12):2453–6.

[77] Wijman CA, Babikian VL, Matjucha IC, et al. Cerebral microembolism in patients with retinal ischemia. Stroke 1998;29(6):1139–43.

[78] Barnett HJ. Delayed cerebral ischemic episodes distal to occlusion of major cerebral arteries. Neurology 1978;28(8):769–74.

[79] Barnett HJ, Peerless SJ, Kaufmann JC. "Stump" on internal carotid artery—a source for further cerebral embolic ischemia. Stroke 1978;9(5): 448–56.

[80] Finklestein S, Kleinman GM, Cuneo R, et al. Delayed stroke following carotid occlusion. Neurology 1980;30(1):84–8.

[81] Georgiadis D, Grosset DG, Lees KR. Transhemispheric passage of microemboli in patients with unilateral internal carotid artery occlusion. Stroke 1993;24(11):1664–6.

[82] Pugsley W, Klinger L, Paschalis C, et al. The impact of microemboli during cardiopulmonary bypass on neuropsychological functioning. Stroke 1994;25(7):1393–9.

[83] Crawley F, Clifton A, Buckenham T, et al. Comparison of hemodynamic cerebral ischemia and microembolic signals detected during carotid endarterectomy and carotid angioplasty. Stroke 1997;28(12):2460–4.

[84] Rapp JH, Pan XM, Yu B, et al. Cerebral ischemia and infarction from atheroemboli <100 microm in size. Stroke 2003;34(8):1976–80.

[85] Rapp JH, Pan XM, Sharp FR, et al. Atheroemboli to the brain: size threshold for causing acute neuronal cell death. J Vasc Surg 2000;32(1):68–76.

[86] Grigg MJ, Papadakis K, Nicolaides AN, et al. The significance of cerebral infarction and atrophy in patients with amaurosis fugax and transient ischemic attacks in relation to internal carotid artery stenosis: a preliminary report. J Vasc Surg 1988;7(2):215–22.

[87] Norris JW, Zhu CZ. Silent stroke and carotid stenosis. Stroke 1992;23(4):483–5.

[88] Gore I, McCombs HL, Lindquist RL. Observations on the fate of cholesterol emboli. J Atheroscler Res 1964;4:527–35.

[89] Kassirer JP. Atheroembolic renal disease. N Engl J Med 1969;280(15):812–8.

[90] Padayachee TS, Parsons S, Theobold R, et al. The detection of microemboli in the middle cerebral artery during cardiopulmonary bypass: a transcranial Doppler ultrasound investigation using membrane and bubble oxygenators. Ann Thorac Surg 1987;44(3):298–302.

[91] Newman MF, Kirchner JL, Phillips-Bute B, et al. Longitudinal assessment of neurocognitive function after coronary-artery bypass surgery. N Engl J Med 2001;344(6):395–402.

[92] Breteler MM, van Swieten JC, Bots ML, et al. Cerebral white matter lesions, vascular risk factors, and cognitive function in a population-based study: the Rotterdam Study. Neurology 1994; 44(7):1246–52.

[93] Longstreth WT Jr, Manolio TA, Arnold A, et al. Clinical correlates of white matter findings on cranial magnetic resonance imaging of 3301 elderly people. The Cardiovascular Health Study. Stroke 1996;27(8):1274–82.

[94] Skoog I, Lernfelt B, Landahl S, et al. 15-year longitudinal study of blood pressure and dementia. Lancet 1996;347(9009):1141–5.

[95] de Groot JC, de Leeuw FE, Oudkerk M, et al. Cerebral white matter lesions and cognitive function: the Rotterdam Scan Study. Ann Neurol 2000;47(2):145–51.

[96] Bigler ED, Lowry CM, Kerr B, et al. Role of white matter lesions, cerebral atrophy, and APOE on cognition in older persons with and without dementia: the Cache County, Utah, study of memory and aging. Neuropsychology 2003;17(3):339–52.

[97] Gunning-Dixon FM, Raz N. Neuroanatomical correlates of selected executive functions in middle-aged and older adults: a prospective MRI study. Neuropsychologia 2003;41(14): 1929–41.

[98] Burton EJ, Kenny RA, O'Brien J, et al. White matter hyperintensities are associated with impairment of memory, attention, and global cognitive performance in older stroke patients. Stroke 2004;35(6):1270–5.

[99] Tullberg M, Fletcher E, DeCarli C, et al. White matter lesions impair frontal lobe function regardless of their location. Neurology 2004; 63(2):246–53.

[100] Burns JM, Church JA, Johnson DK, et al. White matter lesions are prevalent but differentially related with cognition in aging and early Alzheimer disease. Arch Neurol 2005;62(12): 1870–6.

[101] Price CC, Jefferson AL, Merino JG, et al. Subcortical vascular dementia: integrating neuropsychological and neuroradiologic data. Neurology 2005;65(3):376–82.

[102] Prins ND, van Dijk EJ, den Heijer T, et al. Cerebral small-vessel disease and decline in information processing speed, executive function and memory. Brain 2005;128(Pt 9):2034–41.

[103] Au R, Massaro JM, Wolf PA, et al. Association of white matter hyperintensity volume with decreased cognitive functioning: the Framingham Heart Study. Arch Neurol 2006;63(2):246–50.

[104] Nordahl CW, Ranganath C, Yonelinas AP, et al. White matter changes compromise prefrontal cortex function in healthy elderly individuals. J Cogn Neurosci 2006;18(3):418–29.

[105] Boone KB, Miller BL, Lesser IM, et al. Neuropsychological correlates of white-matter lesions in healthy elderly subjects. A threshold effect. Arch Neurol 1992;49(5):549–54.

[106] de Groot JC, de Leeuw FE, Breteler MM. Cognitive correlates of cerebral white matter changes. J Neural Transm Suppl 1998;53:41–67.

[107] Brott T, Tomsick T, Feinberg W, et al. Baseline silent cerebral infarction in the Asymptomatic Carotid Atherosclerosis Study. Stroke 1994; 25(6):1122–9.

[108] Spangler KM, Challa VR, Moody DM, et al. Arteriolar tortuosity of the white matter in aging and hypertension. A microradiographic study. J Neuropathol Exp Neurol 1994;53(1):22–6.

[109] Orlandi G, Parenti G, Bertolucci A, et al. Silent cerebral microembolism in asymptomatic and

symptomatic carotid artery stenoses of low and high degree. Eur Neurol 1997;38(1):39–43.

[110] Vermeer SE, Prins ND, den Heijer T, et al. Silent brain infarcts and the risk of dementia and cognitive decline. N Engl J Med 2003;348(13): 1215–22.

[111] Bernick C, Kuller L, Dulberg C, et al. Silent MRI infarcts and the risk of future stroke: the Cardiovascular Health Study. Neurology 2001;57(7): 1222–9.

[112] Mosley TH Jr, Knopman DS, Catellier DJ, et al. Cerebral MRI findings and cognitive functioning: the Atherosclerosis Risk in Communities Study. Neurology 2005;64(12):2056–62.

[113] Longstreth WT Jr, Bernick C, Manolio TA, et al. Lacunar infarcts defined by magnetic resonance imaging of 3660 elderly people: the Cardiovascular Health Study. Arch Neurol 1998;55(9): 1217–25.

[114] Fernando MS, Ince PG. Vascular pathologies and cognition in a population-based cohort of elderly people. J Neurol Sci 2004;226(1–2):13–7.

[115] Schmidt R, Ropele S, Enzinger C, et al. White matter lesion progression, brain atrophy, and cognitive decline: the Austrian Stroke Prevention Study. Ann Neurol 2005;58(4):610–6.

[116] Manschot SM, Brands AM, van der Grond J, et al. Brain magnetic resonance imaging correlates of impaired cognition in patients with type 2 diabetes. Diabetes 2006;55(4):1106–13.

[117] Gold G, Kovari E, Herrmann FR, et al. Cognitive consequences of thalamic, basal ganglia, and deep white matter lacunes in brain aging and dementia. Stroke 2005;36(6):1184–8.

[118] Ohta H, Nishikawa H, Kimura H, et al. Chronic cerebral hypoperfusion by permanent internal carotid ligation produces learning impairment without brain damage in rats. Neuroscience 1997;79(4):1039–50.

[119] Ni J, Ohta H, Matsumoto K, et al. Progressive cognitive impairment following chronic cerebral hypoperfusion induced by permanent occlusion of bilateral carotid arteries in rats. Brain Res 1994;653(1–2):231–6.

[120] Pappas BA, de la Torre JC, Davidson CM, et al. Chronic reduction of cerebral blood flow in the adult rat: late-emerging CA1 cell loss and memory dysfunction. Brain Res 1996;708(1–2): 50–8.

[121] Tanaka K, Ogawa N, Asanuma M, et al. Relationship between cholinergic dysfunction and discrimination learning disabilities in Wistar rats following chronic cerebral hypoperfusion. Brain Res 1996;729(1):55–65.

[122] Nanri M, Miyake H, Murakami Y, et al. Chronic cerebral hypoperfusion-induced neuropathological changes in rats. Nihon Shinkei Seishin Yakurigaku Zasshi 1998;18(5):181–8.

[123] Wang LM, Han YF, Tang XC. Huperzine A improves cognitive deficits caused by chronic cerebral hypoperfusion in rats. Eur J Pharmacol 2000;398(1):65–72.

[124] Sopala M, Danysz W. Chronic cerebral hypoperfusion in the rat enhances age-related deficits in spatial memory. J Neural Transm 2001; 108(12):1445–56.

[125] Neto CJ, Paganelli RA, Benetoli A, et al. Permanent 3-stage, 4-vessel occlusion as a model of chronic and progressive brain hypoperfusion in rats: a neurohistological and behavioral analysis. Behav Brain Res 2005;160(2): 312–22.

[126] de la Torre JC, Saunders J, Fortin T, et al. Return of ATP/PCr and EEG after 75 min of global brain ischemia. Brain Res 1991;542(1): 71–6.

[127] de la Torre JC, Fortin T, Park GA, et al. Chronic cerebrovascular insufficiency induces dementia-like deficits in aged rats. Brain Res 1992;582(2): 186–95.

[128] de la Torre JC, Fortin T, Park GA, et al. Aged but not young rats develop metabolic, memory deficits after chronic brain ischaemia. Neurol Res 1992;14(Suppl 2):177–80.

[129] Astrup J, Siesjo BK, Symon L. Thresholds in cerebral ischemia—the ischemic penumbra. Stroke 1981;12(6):723–5.

[130] Astrup J, Symon L, Branston NM, et al. Cortical evoked potential and extracellular K+ and H+ at critical levels of brain ischemia. Stroke 1977; 8(1):51–7.

[131] Branston NM, Strong AJ, Symon L. Extracellular potassium activity, evoked potential and tissue blood flow. Relationships during progressive ischaemia in baboon cerebral cortex. J Neurol Sci 1977;32(3):305–21.

[132] Odano I, Miyashita K, Minoshima S, et al. A potential use of a 123I-labelled benzodiazepine receptor antagonist as a predictor of neuronal cell viability: comparisons with 14C-labelled 2-deoxyglucose autoradiography and histopathological examination. Nucl Med Commun 1995;16(6):443–6.

[133] de la Torre JC, Fortin T, Park GA, et al. Brain blood flow restoration 'rescues' chronically damaged rat CA1 neurons. Brain Res 1993; 623(1):6–15.

[134] de la Torre JC, Fortin T. Partial or global rat brain ischemia: the SCOT model. Brain Res Bull 1991;26(3):365–72.

[135] Marshall RS, Lazar RM, Pile-Spellman J, et al. Recovery of brain function during induced cerebral hypoperfusion. Brain 2001;124(Pt 6): 1208–17.

[136] Fisher M. Characterizing the target of acute stroke therapy. Stroke 1997;28(4):866–72.

ELSEVIER
SAUNDERS

NEUROIMAGING
CLINICS
OF NORTH AMERICA

Neuroimag Clin N Am 17 (2007) 325–336

Extracranial Stenosis: Endovascular Treatment

Yince Loh, MD*, Gary R. Duckwiler, MD

- Indications
  - *Patients with normal risk*
  - *High-risk patients*
  - *Current recommendations*
- Other considerations
  - *Neurologic considerations*
- *Anatomic considerations*
- *Medical considerations*
- Imaging
- Technique
- Special situations
- Acknowledgments
- References

Stroke is the third-leading cause of death in the United States [1]. It occurs in almost 700,000 people per year and cost an estimated $57.9 billion in 2006 [1–3]. Atherosclerotic disease is the cause of one third of these strokes, with more than one half of these stenoses being extracranial in location [4,5]. Carotid stenoses are usually unifocal and 90% occur within 2 cm of the carotid bulb [6]. Stenoses amenable to revascularization are the topic of this article.

Currently, carotid endarterectomy (CEA) accounts for 117,000 surgical revascularizations per year, whereas carotid angioplasty and stenting (CAS) are performed less than 10,000 times annually [1]. Endovascular therapy for extracranial carotid stenoses has become an increasingly attractive alternative to surgery. Much of this interest is fueled by advances in technology and technique. Similarly, knowledge of the natural history of lesions treated by endovascular means, and the immediate peri-procedural complications of intervention, have contributed greatly to the interest in minimally invasive techniques.

Advances in endovascular interventional techniques and devices have been rapid. The development

and improvement of distal embolic protection devices (EPDs) and rapid exchange systems allow the endovascular operator rapid and safe access to the carotid lesion. The temporary proximal carotid occlusion required for endarterectomy is now avoidable when using endovascular techniques. Because extracranial carotid disease often occurs in the face of systemic disease, the surgical risk to these patients can be high [7,8]. The minimal invasiveness of CAS makes it an option for these high-risk patients, much in the way coronary angioplasty has become a viable alternative to bypass surgery. Shorter hospital stays, shorter procedural and carotid occlusion times, and freedom from general anesthesia all contribute to the theoretic decrease in procedural risk.

Indications

One of the major difficulties in CAS has been establishing a consensus on the clinical indications for treatment. Endarterectomy became the basis of treatment after the North American Symptomatic Carotid Endarterectomy Trial (NASCET) [9], the

David Geffen School of Medicine at UCLA, Division of Interventional Neuroradiology, 10833 Le Conte Avenue, BL-133 CHS, Los Angeles, CA 90095, USA
* Corresponding author.
E-mail address: yloh@mednet.ucla.edu (Y. Loh).

1052-5149/07/$ – see front matter © 2007 Elsevier Inc. All rights reserved.
neuroimaging.theclinics.com

doi:10.1016/j.nic.2007.03.004

European Carotid Surgery Trial (ECST) [10,11], and the Asymptomatic Carotid Atherosclerotic Study (ACAS) [12] in the 1990s. In the past, many endovascular trials adopted ECST and ACAS exclusion criteria as the basis for inclusion in endovascular trials. As a result, most practitioners had adopted only those criteria as clinical indicators for treatment, until the last several years.

Patients with normal risk

In the normal surgical risk population, the NASCET investigators demonstrated that endarterectomy for high-grade symptomatic carotid stenosis (70%–99%) was better than medical management [9,13]. The absolute risk of major or fatal ipsilateral stroke at 2 years was reduced by 10% by endarterectomy. Since the publication of this data in 1991, the clinical indications for endarterectomy have evolved. The ECST demonstrated that CEA provided benefit in patients with symptomatic lesions greater than 50%. As a result, endarterectomy is performed on this group of normal-risk patients in most clinical vascular surgery practices. In addition, many patients who would have been considered at higher surgical risk (see later discussion) according to ACAS and NASCET criteria are now undergoing endarterectomy, according to Medicare analysis [14,15].

The indications for treating asymptomatic carotid lesions are not as clear-cut. The authors of ACAS demonstrated that asymptomatic lesions greater than 60% benefited from endarterectomy as long as the overall surgical risk was less than 3%. The study design has been criticized for the exclusion of patients with comorbidities, who would have otherwise done poorly. Thus, the population selected was not representative of the patient routinely treated with endarterectomy in clinical practice [16] or his/her operative mortality [17,18]. Another major criticism is that the data may be outdated with regards to advances in medical management, such as more effective antiplatelets and statins [19].

For normal-risk patients, no data suggest CAS is equivalent to CEA in either symptomatic or asymptomatic patients. This field is a topic of ongoing study and debate. Two highly publicized studies attempted to prove that CAS is not inferior to CEA, but failed to do so. Both studies used a noninferiority design, which has the advantage of requiring less numbers than a standard comparison. In the EVA-3S trial, the investigators compared CEA to CAS in symptomatic severe carotid stenosis in normal-risk patients [20]. The study was stopped early because of increased 30-day risks of stroke or death in the CAS group and the inability to enroll the numbers needed to power a study proving equivalence. In

the SPACE trial, the investigators failed to prove noninferiority in normal-risk patients who had moderate-to-severe stenosis. Although the study was not stopped early, they also concluded that they could not enroll the numbers needed to prove equivalence [21]. Although both studies failed to show noninferiority, readers should be cautioned not to interpret the data to suggest that CEA is, in fact, superior to CAS. Ultimately, a large, randomized trial, such as the National Institutes of Health–funded Carotid Revascularization Endarterectomy versus Stent Trial (CREST), is needed to power a true comparison [22,23].

High-risk patients

The issue of the best treatment modality for high-risk patients who have symptomatic stenosis is also a topic of ongoing study and debate. As mentioned earlier, the ECST and ACAS exclusion criteria formed the basis of inclusion in CAS trials, mainly patients with high surgical risk. In total, only three prospective studies analyzed CAS outcomes using each of the three stents currently approved by the Food and Drug Administration [8]. Of these, only one was a randomized clinical trial, the Stenting and Angioplasty with Protection in Patients at High Risk for Endarterectomy (SAPPHIRE). This study is the only randomized clinical trial comparing CAS with CEA in high-risk patients. Its inclusion criteria, asymptomatic lesions greater than 80% and symptomatic lesions greater than 50% in high-risk patients, resulted in the current reimbursement authorization by the Centers for Medicare and Medicaid Services (CMS), and are the basis for ongoing trial registries (Box 3). This authorization, in turn, has made its impact on patient selection for treatment in clinical practice. The 1998 American Heart

---

Box 1:   Centers for Medicare and Medicaid Services reimbursement criteria for carotid angioplasty and stenting

If high surgical risk and symptomatic with stenosis of

>70%: authorized[a]
50%–69%: must be enrolled in category B IDE clinical trials or postapproval study[b]

If high surgical risk and asymptomatic with stenosis of

≥80%: must be enrolled in category B IDE clinical trials or postapproval study[b]

[a] Coverage limited to Food and Drug Administration–approved devices.

[b] as a routine cost per Medicare National Coverage Determinations Manuals 20.7 and 310.1, Regulation 42 CFR 405.201sz.

Association (AHA) expert consensus panel [26] defined the medical and anatomic conditions considered risk factors associated with increased complications after CEA (**Box 2**), which have been adopted since, for purposes of CMS reimbursement.

As mentioned earlier, a large, prospective, randomized trial comparing CEA with CAS is needed. The National Institutes of Health–funded CREST is ongoing and randomizing 1400 symptomatic, normal-risk patients who have greater than 50% stenosis by angiography or greater than 70% by ultrasound, and 1100 asymptomatic, normal-risk patients who have greater than 60% stenosis by angiography or greater than 70% by ultrasound. The International Carotid Stenting Study (ICSS), also known as CAVATAS-2, is also an ongoing, multicenter, randomized trial with a planned enrollment of 1500 patients [27]. The study plans to compare the two techniques in normal-risk patients who have symptomatic severe stenosis.

Current recommendations

Only recently has expert consensus attempted to clarify the indications for CAS. The document is the American Heart Association/American Stroke Association (AHA/ASA) Recommendations for Revascularization in Symptomatic Patients, (**Box 3**) [28], which recommends CAS only for symptomatic lesions greater than 70% in high-risk patients. As a result, CMS now authorizes reimbursement for high-risk symptomatic patients who have greater than 70% stenosis. It also authorizes reimbursement for high-risk patients who have symptomatic lesions greater than 50% and asymptomatic lesions greater than 80% when enrolled in a Category B investigational device exemption (IDE) clinical trial or postapproval study (see **Box 1**). Ultimately, this reimbursement authorization has become the driving force of patient selection in clinical practice.

Other considerations

Many nuances to an individual's condition may preclude endovascular revascularization, despite meeting the inclusion criteria discussed earlier. In some of these situations, the exclusionary aspect may not become apparent until the patient has presented to the angiography suite and been catheterized. The absolute and relative contraindications can be grouped into neurologic, medical, and anatomic considerations (**Box 4**).

Neurologic considerations

The neurologic considerations relate mostly to long-term quality of life. Because many potential candidates may be older and have long-standing hypertension, some degree of intracranial disease is inevitable. Whether the burden of ischemic white-matter disease is significant enough to impair cognition is unique to that individual. No randomized controlled trials have evaluated the long-term improvement in quality of life in patients who have cognitive impairment. As the degree of cognitive impairment increases, so does the confidence that CAS will not improve functionality or long-term morbidity. Thus, it is reasonable to consider "severe" cognitive functional impairment a contraindication to CAS.

Currently, major stroke within 4 weeks is a relative contraindication. However, acute strokes are sometimes the exception to this rule. These strokes can involve collateral failure or artery-to-artery embolization, and these special circumstances are discussed in detail in the last section.

Anatomic considerations

Anatomic considerations relate to the degree of underlying age-related and chronic hypertensive changes in the vascular system and the structural characteristics of the stenosis. Safe vascular access is required before the start of any angiographic procedure. Chronic hypertensives and vasculopaths are at risk of developing peripheral vascular disease, iliac artery stenoses, and aortic aneurysms. Alternatively, they may have a history of surgical correction for these conditions, both of which may make catheterization difficult or hazardous.

After vascular access is obtained, being able to navigate to the lesion in question can be difficult. Age and chronic hypertension can alter thoracic and cervical vascular anatomy, which makes catheterization difficult. An unwound aorta and

tortuosity of the origins of the innominate and left common carotid arteries may be severe enough to preclude CAS. In certain situations, where takeoff angles are severe, brachial or radial access may be an alternative, particularly in regards to the origin of the right common carotid artery or a bovine origin of the left common carotid. The cervical portions of the common and internal carotid arteries may be tortuous themselves, allowing for navigation of a microguidewire but not the stiffer stent delivery systems. Factors such as the tortuosity of the brachiocephalic system or a type III aortic arch (when the origin of the innominate artery is caudal to the inner inferior curve of the aortic arch) may make it difficult to maintain access with the guiding catheter. Such difficulty may also lead to prolonged EPD deployment time, which has been shown to be an independent risk factor for procedural complications [25].

The morphology of the lesion itself should be analyzed before pursuing CAS. A heavily calcified or circumferential lesion may be a relative contraindication. Because calcification is very resistant to balloon dilatation, the radial force from a self-expanding nitinol stent is also likely to be insufficient. Visible thrombus as a component of an atherosclerotic lesion is also a contraindication. The exception, as discussed in the last section, is acute stroke treatment.

Patients have a lower risk of ipsilateral stroke in the territory of a carotid artery if it is nearly or totally occluded [29,30]. Thus, the presence of a "string sign" by MR angiography or carotid Doppler ultrasonography (DUS) is a relative contraindication. In severe stenoses that may not qualify as near-occlusion, one of the considerations is vessel collapse. If little forward perfusion pressure is seen across a large gradient created by the stenosis, the distal carotid can be collapsed significantly (Fig. 1), which may pose a problem with distal EPD selection. The smallest EPD currently available is 2.0 mm in diameter. If the anteroposterior (AP) dimension is collapsed enough not to accommodate such an EPD, CAS may not be possible and may be hazardous if performed without one. Additionally, should a distal EPD fit properly, it may not be sufficient to protect from distal embolization of debris when the gradient is normalized, forward perfusion pressure is restored, and the normal diameter of the distal vessel is restored, producing a situation where the initial EPD selection is undersized.

Medical considerations

Certain medical conditions exist that may be contraindications to CAS. Renal insufficiency should be evaluated carefully. Postponement of

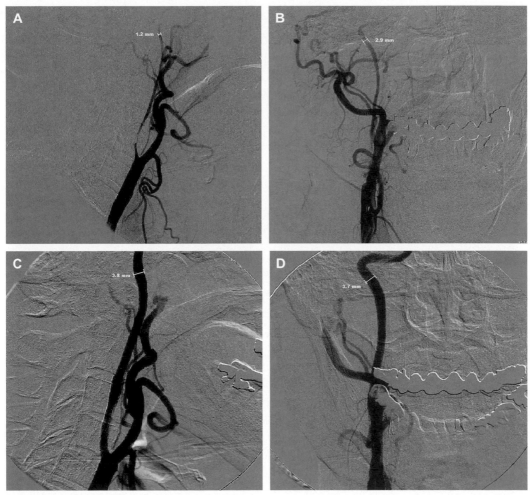

Fig. 1. Distal internal carotid artery collapse can limit EPD selection. The lateral projection digital subtraction angiography (*A*) demonstrates a significantly smaller distal internal carotid artery diameter than the anteroposterior projection (*B*), which ultimately determines the EPD. Following CAS, the diameter of the native vessel with normal perfusion pressure is significantly larger, as seen on lateral (*C*) and anteroposterior (*D*) digital subtraction angiography.

intervention may be required to allow for medical and intravascular volume optimization and to reduce the risk of contrast nephropathy [31]. If CAS is absolutely necessary, the patient and family should be informed of the possibility of impending hemodialysis, which can potentially be lifelong, altering the risk/benefit ratio considerably.

Life expectancy is an important consideration when calculating the risk/benefit ratio for CAS. In asymptomatic patients with a less than 5-year life expectancy or symptomatic patients with a less than 3-year life expectancy, CAS may be contraindicated, based on the ACAS and NASCET data [9,12].

Post-CAS management has adopted cardiology recommendations for antiplatelet therapy to prevent stent luminal thrombosis. Any contraindication to the use of antiplatelets similarly precludes CAS as an option. However, the patient's ability to

tolerate a single agent may be sufficient to proceed. No evidence at this time suggests that the use of double antiplatelet therapy is superior to a single agent in preventing cerebrovascular ischemic events [32], whereas the use of double antiplatelet therapy in preventing endovascular stent restenosis is common in clinical practice [33], but lacking Level I evidence.

Age is a controversial contraindication in carotid revascularization. In observational studies, age older than 80 was an independent risk factor for post-CEA stroke [34]. This age cut-off has also been adapted by the American College of Cardiology as a contraindication to CEA [26]. Although SAPPHIRE did not exclude octogenarians and, in fact, showed fewer complications with CAS than CEA, CREST suspended enrollment of this group because of a higher risk in its lead-in phase of the study [23].

However, the randomized phase of CREST has no age limit, in keeping with the NASCET design. At present, no Level I evidence indicates age older than 80 is a risk factor for post-CAS complications.

Gender is also a controversial topic in the CEA literature. NASCET showed less long-term benefit of surgery for women than men [13], whereas another study showed increased perioperative mortality in women [35]. Subgroup analysis of NASCET data revealed that women had a decreasing benefit with increasing treatment delay from time of initial stroke [36]. To date, however, no conclusive evidence exists that gender affects CAS outcome.

Imaging

Institutions vary in the primary imaging modality used to assess carotid disease. The most common modalities include DUS, MR angiography, CT angiography, and catheter digital subtraction angiography (DSA). Of these, the first is the least invasive, and the last is the most. Each modality has its own advantages and disadvantages.

The modality of choice is dictated by the specialty service requesting or performing the examination. For instance, vascular surgery practices often have their own laboratories that perform DUS simply because it is easy to operate, does not require advanced scheduling, is fairly reproducible, can offer longitudinal comparison, and has the least space requirement of all the modalities.

The best modality has been debated often. DSA remains the gold standard, although it fails to disclose plaque morphology [37] and subtle calcification, one of the contraindications to CAS. Many studies have examined and compared the sensitivities and specificities of each [38,39]. The lack of consensus means the choice is left up to the individual practitioner. The requirements needed to diagnose clinically significant stenosis by each modality are discussed in this section. The standard thus far has been set by the NASCET investigators, although they used angiography for diagnosis. They calculated the percentage of internal carotid artery (ICA) stenosis by comparing the narrowest ICA luminal diameter with the diameter of the normal distal cervical ICA. However, widely used duplex scan criteria for ICA stenosis were developed on the basis of estimated bulb diameter [39].

DUS is probably the most ubiquitous of the carotid imaging techniques. However, investigators have disputed the sole use of ultrasound before selection for endarterectomy [40]. In 2003, the Society of Radiologists in Ultrasound delivered a consensus statement from their conference detailing the requirements for diagnosing stenosis [41]. This consensus required that several criteria be met. All studies should be performed using color Doppler, grayscale, and spectral DUS. The presence of plaque on ultrasonography and ICA peak systolic velocity are the primary factors used. Greater than 50% stenosis is diagnosed when peak systolic velocity is greater than 125 cm/s, and stenosis greater than or equal to 70% when peak systolic velocity is greater than 230 cm/s.

MR angiography using either gadolinium contrast-enhanced or time-of-flight acquisition is a minimally invasive technique that continues to evolve as magnet strengths and postprocessing software continues to improve. Again, NASCET continues to serve as the criteria for measurement. Of these two modalities, contrast-enhanced MR angiography of the neck is widely becoming the preferred method of MR angiography because of its higher image quality, interobserver correlation, and diagnostic reliability [42]. Contrast-enhanced MR angiography of the neck has even been shown to have accurate correlation with DSA [43].

CT angiography of the neck vessels has not proved reliable as a sole methodology in carotid stenosis evaluation. It has been shown to obviate the need for DSA when used in conjunction with DUS [44], although it can fail to demonstrate the lumen accurately within a circumferential calcified plaque [45]. CT angiography is equally useful in conjunction with either contrast-enhanced MR angiography or DUS in the evaluation of carotid stenosis, but it is inaccurate in evaluating asymptomatic severe stenoses as a sole modality [46].

In endovascular therapy for carotid disease, the exact modality used to select a patient for treatment is not entirely irrelevant. It is true that a patient selected in such a way will always undergo DSA before any planned intervention. If the degree of stenosis measured by DSA does not meet clinical indications, the procedure is aborted. However, to avoid performing an unnecessary invasive procedure, the endovascular operator should ensure that the noninvasive images are of good quality and that the technique and measurement criteria are satisfactory.

Technique

Most experts in the field believe that reduction of distal embolization is much more important than achieving a completely normal angiographic result. From this standpoint, the goal of CAS is to cross the stenotic lesion as few times as possible, deploy distal EPD, and dilate the stenotic area without complications.

Generally, carotid catheterization is achieved using the usual angiographic technique, and initial catheter and wire selection depends mostly on the

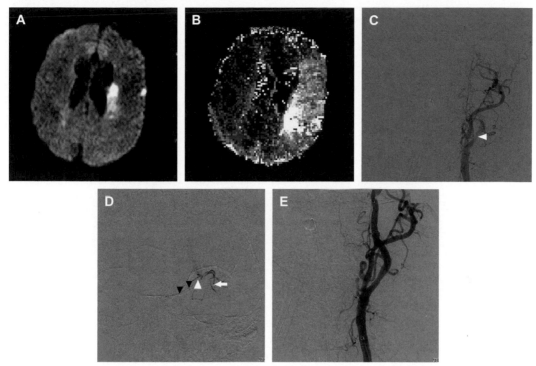

Fig. 2. CAS in the setting of acute artery-to-artery embolization. MR imaging area of diffusion restriction (*A*) is outweighed by the perfusion defect (*B*), suggesting a proximal M1 occlusion, which may necessitate mechanical embolectomy. An AP DSA of the cervical ICA (*C*) shows moderate stenosis (*arrowhead*) but severe perfusion delay, suggesting a large distal clot burden. Superselective AP DSA (*D*) after distal microcatheterization (*black arrowheads*) beyond the M1 occlusion (*arrow*) shows the M1 thrombus (*white arrowhead*). CAS of the cervical ICA lesion (*E*) prevents further thromboembolization or allows safer access for mechanical embolectomy. (Currently, clot retrieval devices are not indicated for use when there is >50% proximal stenosis).

patient's vascular anatomy and the operator's preference. The proximal common carotid artery, or even the external carotid artery, can be selected initially. Once distal positioning has been established, the operator can exchange the diagnostic catheter for either a 6F interventional sheath or an 8F guiding catheter over an exchange wire (both have similar inner luminal diameters, 0.087–0.09 in). With either of these, the distal tip can then be brought into the cervical common carotid artery (CCA).

Heparinization begins once the interventional sheath or guiding catheter is in position. Deployment of a distal EPD occurs next. Proximal EPDs are being used in Europe but are not approved yet in the United States. Thus, only distal EPDs are discussed in this article.

The SPACE [21], ARCHeR [24], and EVA-3S [20] trials showed no statistical difference between CAS with and without EPDs. However, the EVA-3S investigators changed their protocol midstudy to require EPDs based on interim detection of a nonsignificant difference in outcomes. Although no randomized controlled trials compare CAS with and without EPDs, observational studies alone make it unlikely

that future CAS trials will be performed without EPD [47]. Similarly, CMS recommends the use of distal EPDs, and their use dominates clinical practice.

No evidence suggests that one of the two principle types of distal EPD is superior to the other. The first type uses balloon occlusion distally and aspiration of any debris elicited by the intervention before balloon deflation. The second relies on a filter device that permits antegrade flow while capturing debris, then is retrieved together with any debris. The filter EPD trades reliability of debris arrest for preserved antegrade flow and ability to contrast image throughout the procedure. The former carries a risk of balloon-induced injury, whereas the latter runs the risk of filter obstruction and device entrapment within the stent during retrieval. All distal EPDs inherently risk embolization when the stenosis is traversed with the microwire, microcatheter, or EPD deployment system.

Regardless of the distal EPD choice, it is optimal to have the EPD deployed before any other intervention, but a tightly stenotic lesion may not allow passage of the device. Thus, in certain circumstances,

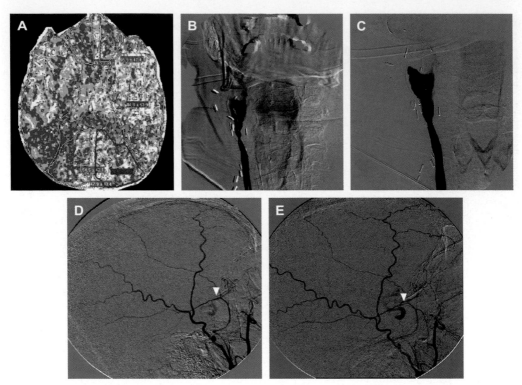

Fig. 3. ECA reperfusion by CAS. A CCA previously treated by CEA and now occluded causes hypoperfusion of the ICA vessels by CT perfusion (*A*). The moderate stenosis of the distal CCA before treatment (*B*) is improved by CAS (*C*). Although intracranial lateral DSA before (*D*) and after (*E*) CAS shows improved collateral filling of the ICA siphon through ophthalmic collaterals (*arrowheads*), the primary purpose was to treat the proximal, flow-limiting CCA stenosis before superior temporal artery to middle cerebral artery (STA-MCA) bypass. The patient did not have an anterior communicating artery and the posterior communicating artery was stenosed.

unprotected dilatation with a 2-mm balloon may be necessary to allow distal access. Distal EPDs are attached to a microwire (usually 0.014 in), over which various new rapid-exchange CAS systems and balloon catheters can be used, allowing an operator to perform the procedure unassisted.

Once distal protection is established, angioplasty typically is used next, as an adjunctive technique to stenting. The initial balloon selection is undersized, relative to the native ICA (a balloon:ICA ratio of 0.5–0.6); the purpose is merely to allow passage of the typically wider profile stent delivery system through the stenotic lesion.

Two types of stents are commonly used in carotid atherosclerotic disease. Nitinol or stainless steel self-expanding stents are typically used in cervical CCA or ICA lesions because they are conformable yet can withstand the impacts of neck rotation or compression. Although no evidence points to nitinol's superiority over stainless steel, operators often choose it because of better deployment predictability. Balloon-expandable coronary stents are commonly used only for intrathoracic CCA or origin lesions.

Following stent deployment, another undersized balloon is used to expand the stent (balloon:ICA ratio

of 0.6–0.8). Minimizing the number of balloon dilatations is essential to minimize the risk of complications and autonomic instability generated by bulb manipulation. Generally, a residual stenosis of 30% to 40% is acceptable because self-expanding Nitinol stents may continue to expand the lumen with time. Heavy or concentric calcification of the plaque may be the primary reason for a residual stenosis, and this calcification generally does not respond to low pressure (≤ 6 atmospheres) balloon dilatation.

Following poststent dilatation, the EPD is retrieved, and the intervention is complete. Care must be taken to ensure that the device is not entrapped by the stent struts as the operator navigates the EPD through the lumen.

Special situations

Some unusual circumstances may require CAS outside the usual clinical indications. These situations usually occur in patients who have concomitant coronary artery disease in need of bypass surgery. A second scenario exists when there is a need to catheterize distal to a stenosed area. Another situation is one where increased collateral flow is

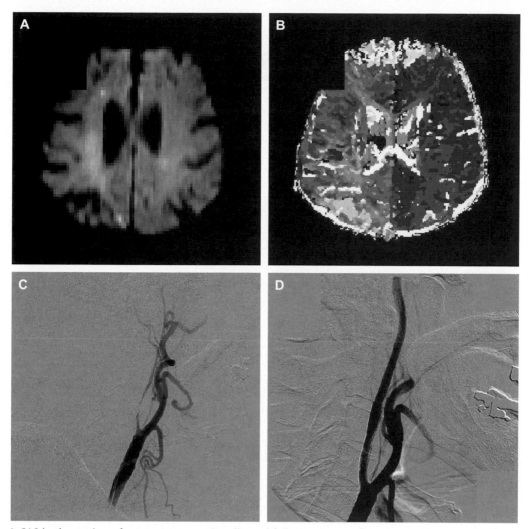

Fig. 4. CAS in the setting of acute symptomatic collateral failure. MR imaging area of diffusion restriction (*A*) is outweighed by the perfusion defect (*B*). Collateral failure from a near-occlusion of the cervical ICA (*C*) shows a near-occlusion. Post-CAS lateral DSA (*D*) was performed without difficulty.

needed, usually in the context of known ICA occlusion.

CAS is a potential precoronary artery bypass graft (CABG) option in treating concomitant coronary artery disease. In the patient who requires coronary artery revascularization, the risk of post-CABG stroke is four times higher when there is a past clinical history of cerebral ischemia, and 10 times higher when there is an asymptomatic carotid stenosis greater than 75% [48]. The current guidelines for CABG [49] recommend that CEA be done before, or concomitant with, coronary revascularization in patients who have asymptomatic stenoses greater than 80% or symptomatic stenoses greater than 50%. Thus, it seems reasonable for patients with this degree of stenosis who do not require urgent CABG to undergo CAS first in a Category B IDE or

postmarketing trial, which requires that coronary revascularization be delayed a minimum of 5 weeks following CAS because of the antiplatelet requirement [22]. In patients who are symptomatic from a stenosis greater than 70%, evidence is sufficient to support performing CAS outside any high-risk registry because the cardiac status alone qualifies as a risk factor for CEA.

The American College of Cardiology Foundation Task Force on Clinical Expert Consensus Documents (ACCF CECD) considers the presence of an intracranial aneurysm or an arteriovenous malformation (AVM) that requires treatment within the distribution of a stenotic carotid a contraindication to CAS. In this situation, augmentation of cerebral perfusion pressure through carotid revascularization may theoretically increase the risk of aneurysm or AVM rupture. However, one study demonstrated that patients who had both carotid stenosis and unruptured intracranial aneurysms did not have subarachnoid hemorrhage after carotid treatment [50]. Thus, if an intracranial aneurysm or AVM requires treatment, the stenosis may need addressing first. Because AVM or aneurysm treatments often require high microcatheter support, more distal sheath or guide catheter placement is necessary. Tandem lesions such as these are not limited to AVMs and aneurysms; they can also include intracranial atherosclerotic disease, acute cerebral embolism, or dural arteriovenous fistulae (Fig. 2).

It is common for patients who have atherosclerotic disease to have multiple stenotic lesions. External carotid disease is often discovered incidentally during evaluation or treatment of an internal or common carotid stenosis, but left alone. The exceptions to the rule are when a longstanding ICA occlusion has led to collaterals supplied by the external carotid artery (ECA), or when a planned ECA-ICA bypass necessitates adequate ECA perfusion (Fig. 3). Should such an ECA develop a flow-limiting stenosis, the brain may become ischemic. In these situations, ECA stenting may be indicated. The technique of ECA stenting is no different than in the ICA, with the exception that most operators consider the ECA a higher-risk vessel for dissection. Care should also be taken to ensure whenever possible that the origin of the ECA branch felt to be the primary source of collateral flow is not obstructed by the stent.

In the setting of acute stroke, treatment revolves around preserving the tissue at risk from further ischemia, the so-called "ischemic penumbra" [51]. Although major stroke within 4 weeks is considered a relative contraindication, CAS may be necessary in the acute setting. Two circumstances that may result in an ischemic penumbra and may require CAS are acute artery-to-artery embolus and collateral failure. In the former, a longstanding carotid stenosis may acutely thrombose or reach a degree of severity that exceeds the cerebrovascular reserve of the leptomeningeal collaterals. Emergent CAS may be the only method to restore cerebral perfusion and preserve the penumbra (Fig. 4). In the latter, artery-to-artery embolization from a carotid lesion may require CAS to provide distal access for follow-on mechanical embolectomy (see Fig. 2). In fact, a proximal stenosis of greater than 50% is considered a contraindication to the use of a clot retrieval device [52].

Acknowledgments

The authors wish to thank Jordan Ziegler, MD, for his assistance in preparing the boxes for this article.

References

[1] American Heart Association. Heart disease and stroke statistics—2006 update. Circulation 2006;113:e85–151.

[2] Kleindorfer D, Panagos P, Pancioli A, et al. Incidence and short-term prognosis of transient ischemic attack in a population-based study. Stroke 2005;36(4):720–3.

[3] Mas JL, Chatellier G, Beyssen B. EVA-3S Investigators. Carotid angioplasty and stenting with and without cerebral protection: clinical alert from the Endarterectomy Versus Angioplasty in patients with Symptomatic Severe carotid Stenosis (EVA-3S) trial. Stroke 2004;35(1):e18–20.

[4] Bamford J, Sandercock P, Dennis M, et al. Classification and natural history of clinically identifiable subtypes of cerebral infarction. Lancet 1991; 337(8756):1521–6.

[5] Gorelick PB. Distribution of atherosclerotic cerebrovascular lesions. Effects of age, race, and sex. Stroke 1993;24(12 Suppl):I16–9.

[6] Mohr JP, Gautier J. Internal carotid disease. In: Barnett HJM, Mohr JP, Stein B, et al, editors. Stroke: pathophysiology, diagnosis, and management. Philadelphia: Churchill Livingstone; 1998. p. 355–400.

[7] Endovascular versus surgical treatment in patients with carotid stenosis in the Carotid and Vertebral Artery Transluminal Angioplasty Study (CAVATAS): a randomised trial. Lancet 2001; 357(9270):1729–37.

[8] Yadav JS, Wholey MH, Kuntz RE, et al. Stenting and Angioplasty with Protection in Patients at High Risk for Endarterectomy Investigators. Protected carotid-artery stenting versus endarterectomy in high-risk patients. N Engl J Med 2004; 351(15):1493–501.

[9] Beneficial effect of carotid endarterectomy in symptomatic patients with high-grade carotid stenosis. North American Symptomatic Carotid Endarterectomy Trial Collaborators. N Engl J Med 1991;325(7):445–53.

[10] MRC European Carotid Surgery Trial: interim results for symptomatic patients with severe (70–99%) or with mild (0–29%) carotid stenosis. European Carotid Surgery Trialists' Collaborative Group. Lancet 1991;337(8752):1235–43.

[11] Randomised trial of endarterectomy for recently symptomatic carotid stenosis: final results of the MRC European Carotid Surgery Trial (ECST). Lancet 1998;351(9113):1379–87.

[12] Endarterectomy for asymptomatic carotid artery stenosis. Executive Committee for the Asymptomatic Carotid Atherosclerosis Study. JAMA 1995;273(18):1421–8.

[13] Barnett HJ, Taylor DW, Eliasziw M, et al. Benefit of carotid endarterectomy in patients with symptomatic moderate or severe stenosis. North American Symptomatic Carotid Endarterectomy Trial Collaborators. N Engl J Med 1998; 339(20):1415–25.

[14] Mozes G. High-risk carotid endarterectomy. Semin Vasc Surg 2005;18(2):61–8.

[15] Weiss JS, Dumas P, Cha C, et al. Safety of carotid endarterectomy in a high-risk population: lessons from the VA and Connecticut. J Am Coll Surg 2006;203(3):277–82.

[16] Barnett HJ, Eliasziw M, Meldrum HE, et al. Do the facts and figures warrant a 10-fold increase in the performance of carotid endarterectomy on asymptomatic patients? Neurology 1996; 46(3):603–8.

[17] Hsia DC, Moscoe LM, Krushat WM. Epidemiology of carotid endarterectomy among Medicare beneficiaries: 1985–1996 update. Stroke 1998; 29(2):346–50.

[18] Wennberg DE, Lucas FL, Birkmeyer JD, et al. Variation in carotid endarterectomy mortality in the Medicare population: trial hospitals, volume, and patient characteristics. JAMA 1998;279(16): 1278–81.

[19] Chaturvedi S. Should the multicenter carotid endarterectomy trials be repeated? Arch Neurol 2003;60:774–5.

[20] Mas JL, Chatellier G, Beyssen B, et al. EVA-3S Investigators. Endarterectomy versus stenting in patients with symptomatic severe carotid stenosis. N Engl J Med 2006;355(16):1660–71.

[21] Ringleb PA, Allenberg J, Bruckmann H, et al. SPACE Collaborative Group. 30 day results from the SPACE trial of stent-protected angioplasty versus carotid endarterectomy in symptomatic patients: a randomised non-inferiority trial. Lancet 2006;368(9543):1239–47.

[22] ACCF/SCAI/SVMB/SIR/ASITN Clinical Expert Consensus Document on Carotid Stenting. A report of the American College of Cardiology Foundation Task Force on Clinical Expert Consensus Documents. J Am Coll Cardiol 2007;49: 126–70.

[23] Hobson RW 2nd, Howard VJ, Roubin GS, et al. CREST Investigators. Carotid artery stenting is associated with increased complications in octogenarians: 30-day stroke and death rates in the CREST lead-in phase. J Vasc Surg 2004;40(6): 1106–11.

[24] Gray WA, Hopkins LN, Yadav S, et al. ARCHeR Trial Collaborators. Protected carotid stenting in high-surgical-risk patients: the ARCHeR results. J Vasc Surg 2006;44(2):258–68.

[25] Safian RD, Bresnahan JF, Jaff MR, et al. CREATE Pivotal Trial Investigators. Protected carotid stenting in high-risk patients with severe carotid artery stenosis. J Am Coll Cardiol 2006;47(12): 2384–9.

[26] Biller J, Feinberg WM, Castaldo JE, et al. Guidelines for carotid endarterectomy: a statement for healthcare professionals from a special writing group of the Stroke Council, American Heart Association. Circulation 1998;97(5):501–9.

[27] Featherstone RL, Brown MM, Coward LJ. ICSS Investigators. International carotid stenting study: protocol for a randomised clinical trial comparing carotid stenting with endarterectomy in symptomatic carotid artery stenosis. Cerebrovasc Dis 2004;18(1):69–74.

[28] Sacco RL, Adams R, Albers G, et al. American Heart Association/American Stroke Association Council on Stroke; Council on Cardiovascular Radiology and Intervention; American Academy of Neurology. Guidelines for prevention of stroke in patients with ischemic stroke or transient ischemic attack: a statement for healthcare professionals from the American Heart Association/American Stroke Association Council on Stroke: co-sponsored by the Council on Cardiovascular Radiology and Intervention: the American Academy of Neurology affirms the value of this guideline. Stroke 2006;37(2):577–617.

[29] Morgenstern LB, Fox AJ, Sharpe BL, et al. The risks and benefits of carotid endarterectomy in patients with near occlusion of the carotid artery. North American Symptomatic Carotid Endarterectomy Trial (NASCET) Group. Neurology 1997; 48(4):911–5.

[30] Rothwell PM, Warlow CP. Low risk of ischemic stroke in patients with reduced internal carotid artery lumen diameter distal to severe symptomatic carotid stenosis: cerebral protection due to low poststenotic flow? On behalf of the European Carotid Surgery Trialists' Collaborative Group. Stroke 2000;31(3):622–30.

[31] Barrett BJ, Parfrey PS. Clinical practice. Preventing nephropathy induced by contrast medium. N Engl J Med 2006;354(4):379–86.

[32] Diener HC, Bogousslavsky J, Brass LM, et al. MATCH investigators. Aspirin and clopidogrel compared with clopidogrel alone after recent ischaemic stroke or transient ischaemic attack in high-risk patients (MATCH): randomised, double-blind, placebo-controlled trial. Lancet 2004; 364(9431):331–7.

[33] Holmes DR Jr. Antiplatelet therapy after percutaneous coronary intervention. Cerebrovasc Dis 2006;21(Suppl 1):25–34.

[34] Bond R, Rerkasem K, Rothwell PM. Systematic review of the risks of carotid endarterectomy in relation to the clinical indication for and timing of surgery. Stroke 2003;34(9):2290–301.

[35] Alamowitch S, Eliasziw M, Barnett HJ, North American Symptomatic Carotid Endarterectomy Trial (NASCET); ASA Trial Group; Carotid Endarterectomy (ACE) Trial Group. The risk and benefit of endarterectomy in women with symptomatic internal carotid artery disease. Stroke 2005;36(1):27–31.

[36] Rothwell PM, Eliasziw M, Gutnikov SA, et al. Sex difference in the effect of time from symptoms to surgery on benefit from carotid endarterectomy for transient ischemic attack and nondisabling stroke. Stroke 2004;35(12):2855–61.

[37] Kagawa R, Moritake K, Shima T, et al. Validity of B-mode ultrasonographic findings in patients undergoing carotid endarterectomy in comparison

with angiographic and clinicopathologic features. Stroke 1996;27(4):700–5.

[38] Eliasziw M, Rankin RN, Fox AJ, et al. Accuracy and prognostic consequences of ultrasonography in identifying severe carotid artery stenosis. North American Symptomatic Carotid Endarterectomy Trial (NASCET) Group. Stroke 1995; 26(10):1747–52.

[39] Moneta GL, Edwards JM, Chitwood RW, et al. Correlation of North American Symptomatic Carotid Endarterectomy Trial (NASCET) angiographic definition of 70% to 99% internal carotid artery stenosis with duplex scanning. J Vasc Surg 1993;17(1):152–7.

[40] Collins P, McKay I, Rajagoplan S, et al. Is carotid duplex scanning sufficient as the sole investigation prior to carotid endarterectomy? Br J Radiol 2005;78(935):1034–7.

[41] Grant EG, Benson CB, Moneta GL, et al. Carotid artery stenosis: gray-scale and Doppler US diagnosis–Society of Radiologists in Ultrasound Consensus Conference. Radiology 2003;229(2):340–6.

[42] Mitra D, Connolly D, Jenkins S, et al. Comparison of image quality, diagnostic confidence and interobserver variability in contrast enhanced MR angiography and 2D time of flight angiography in evaluation of carotid stenosis. Br J Radiol 2006;79(939):201–7.

[43] Remonda L, Senn P, Barth A, et al. Contrast-enhanced 3D MR angiography of the carotid artery: comparison with conventional digital subtraction angiography. AJNR Am J Neuroradiol 2002; 23(2):213–9.

[44] Herzig R, Burval S, Krupka B, et al. Comparison of ultrasonography, CT angiography, and digital subtraction angiography in severe carotid stenoses. Eur J Neurol 2004;11(11):774–81.

[45] Hirai T, Korogi Y, Ono K, et al. Prospective evaluation of suspected stenoocclusive disease of the intracranial artery: combined MR angiography and CT angiography compared with digital subtraction angiography. AJNR Am J Neuroradiol 2002;23(1):93–101.

[46] Nonent M, Serfaty JM, Nighoghossian N, et al. CARMEDAS Study Group. Concordance rate differences of 3 noninvasive imaging techniques to measure carotid stenosis in clinical routine practice: results of the CARMEDAS multicenter study. Stroke 2004;35(3):682–6.

[47] Kastrup A, Groschel K, Krapf H, et al. Early outcome of carotid angioplasty and stenting with and without cerebral protection devices: a systematic review of the literature. Stroke 2003; 34(3):813–9.

[48] Naylor AR, Mehta Z, Rothwell PM, et al. Carotid artery disease and stroke during coronary artery bypass: a critical review of the literature. Eur J Vasc Endovasc Surg 2002;23(4):283–94.

[49] Eagle KA, Guyton RA, Davidoff R, et al. American College of Cardiology; American Heart Association. ACC/AHA 2004 guideline update for coronary artery bypass graft surgery: a report of the American College of Cardiology/American Heart Association Task Force on Practice Guidelines (Committee to Updae the 1999 Guidelines for Coronary Artery Bypass Graft Surgery). Circulation 2004;110(14):e340–437.

[50] Ballotta E, Da Giau G, Manara R, et al. Extracranial severe carotid stenosis and incidental intracranial aneurysms. Ann Vasc Surg 2006;20(1): 5–8.

[51] Kidwell CS, Alger JR, Saver JL. Beyond mismatch: evolving paradigms in imaging the ischemic penumbra with multimodal magnetic resonance imaging. Stroke 2003;34(11):2729–35.

[52] Smith WS, Sung G, Starkman S, et al. MERCI Trial Investigators. Safety and efficacy of mechanical embolectomy in acute ischemic stroke: results of the MERCI trial. Stroke 2005;36(7): 1432–8.

NEUROIMAGING CLINICS OF NORTH AMERICA

Neuroimag Clin N Am 17 (2007) 337–353

Techniques of Carotid Angioplasty and Stenting

Christopher J. Moran, MD*, DeWitte T. Cross, III, MD,
Colin P. Derdeyn, MD

In the article by Loh and Duckwiler, the authors presented the rationale for selecting patients for carotid artery revascularization. They discussed the indications for the procedure and the ensuing benefits, and mentioned the techniques of carotid endarterectomy (CEA) and carotid angioplasty and stenting (CAS). In this article, the authors discuss the decision process leading to choices in the materials and techniques used in CAS, the procedure itself, and the results. The goal of CAS is restoration of a near-normal lumen. The angioplasty expands the lumen in the diseased stenotic carotid artery, and the stent prevents recoil and restrains protruding intima and plaque, thereby maintaining the just-restored lumen.

Preparation

One of the most important steps for any successful procedure is preparation. For CAS, the clinical and imaging evaluation of the patient to determine the suitability of the procedure is essential. The symptomatology determines whether a patient will be low or high risk, or is perhaps not even a candidate for CAS.

The patient's imaging must be reviewed to evaluate both the vasculature and the intracranial contents. If the patient is symptomatic, it is important to determine that the symptoms are caused by ischemia, rather than something else. A recent CT or MR image will detect an infarction or hemorrhage while excluding other processes such as a tumor. Evidence of an infarction may also determine the timing of the procedure. Large areas of damage may lead to hemorrhagic conversion when the supplying carotid artery patency is restored. If the patient has not recovered significantly, or if the infarct volume by imaging is more than one third the territory of the stenotic carotid distribution,

Washington University School of Medicine, Mallinckrodt Institute of Radiology, Department of Neurology and Neurological Surgery, 510 South Kingshighway Blvd., St. Louis, MO 63110, USA
* Corresponding author.
E-mail address: moranc@wustl.edu (C.J. Moran).

1052-5149/07/$ – see front matter © 2007 Elsevier Inc. All rights reserved.
neuroimaging.theclinics.com

doi:10.1016/j.nic.2007.03.003

the authors usually perform angioplasty and stenting 1 month after the incident. This waiting period seems to allow the injured vasculature and brain to heal sufficiently to lessen the risks of hemorrhage after revascularization. The risk of this delay is that the patient may have further ischemic events despite antiplatelet agents. In fact, the tightly stenotic carotid artery may even occlude during the waiting period. In the NASCET study, the nearly occluded ("string sign") symptomatic patients seemed to do reasonably well with medical therapy, with a 1.7% cerebrovascular accident (CVA) rate at 1 month that increased to 11.1% at 1 year, and those undergoing CEA had a stroke rate of 6.3% [1]. Of course, as yet no data exist on angioplasty and stenting in these patients.

During the clinical evaluation, the interventionalist can determine the patient's ability to cooperate. Most procedures are performed with conscious sedation, but some patients may have difficulty cooperating when sedated. In addition, the patient must be able to sustain an open airway while supine under normal (unchallenged) circumstances. Patients who have a history of a contrast allergy should be premedicated with prednisone, 50 mg, by mouth every 6 hours for three doses ending 1 hour before the procedure; just before the procedure, diphenhydramine, 25 mg IV, and an H2 blocker such as cimetidine, 300 mg IV, will prevent and lessen adverse contrast reactions in allergic patients. In cases of severe contrast reactions, intubation for airway control can prevent the respiratory effects of laryngospasm or bronchospasm. Assessment of the patient's renal function will also assist in the selection of an appropriate contrast agent (non-ionic isosmolar) (Visipaque, Amersham PLC, Little Chalfont, Buckinghamshire, UK) for those at risk for the development or worsening of renal failure. In these circumstances, administration of a bicarbonate drip (3 amps bicarbonate in 1 L normal saline at 3 mL/kg for 1 hour before the procedure and 1 mL/kg during the procedure and for 6 hours afterwards) may lessen the incidence of postprocedural renal failure. In addition, the administration of n-acetylcysteine, 600 mg by mouth twice daily the day before and the day of the procedure, may be helpful.

Antiplatelet agents are initiated 5 days before elective procedures: 325 mg of aspirin and 75 mg of clopidogrel bisulphate daily. If the patient has gastrointestinal upset, enteric-coated aspirin can be substituted. For more urgent situations, the patient can be loaded with 300 to 450 mg of clopidogrel bisulphate several hours before the procedure. Intravenous IIb/IIIa inhibitors seem to increase the risk of intracranial hemorrhage and are not recommended for routine CAS [2].

If an arteriogram was performed previously, review of it will demonstrate the aortic arch, the target carotid artery in the neck, and the blood supply to the ipsilateral cerebral hemisphere. The degree of elongation of the aortic arch will help to determine the likelihood of success of a transfemoral approach or the need for an alternative transbrachial or transradial puncture. If the line of origin of the brachiocephalic vessels arises parallel to the upper convexity of the aortic arch (type I aortic arch), the desired carotid artery may be selected using the transfemoral approach with almost no difficulty (Fig. 1). Similarly, if the brachiocephalic vessels arise from the aortic arch between the outer and inner convexities of the aortic arch (type II aortic arch), selecting the desired vessel will be only slightly more difficult (Fig. 2). It is only with the type III aortic arch, where the innominate artery arises below the level of the inner convexity of the aorta, that catheterizing the innominate artery, right common carotid artery, or left common carotid arteries is difficult (Fig. 3). In this instance, it may be difficult to exchange the diagnostic catheter for a guiding catheter or long sheath. Origin of the left common carotid artery from the innominate artery (the so—called "bovine arch") may cause problems for selective catheterization, similar to the type III aortic arch. In these two situations, the transbrachial or transradial approach may be appropriate. (All the authors' CAS procedures have been performed transfemorally.) The direct carotid approach should be used only in patients who are non-CEA candidates and have high lesions and no other access. In these patients, the access site is closed operatively so that the carotid artery is not compressed in an attempt at hemostasis. Successful hemostasis is essential with the direct carotid approach because hematoma formation may compromise the airway. Finally, the carotid artery itself is evaluated because tortuosity of the common carotid artery may cause problems for catheterization. Tortuosity of the internal carotid artery may alter the choice and placement of an embolic protection device (EPD) and the type and site of the stent to be deployed, and even preclude performance of the procedure itself if there are extreme elongation and loops in the carotid artery at or near the treatment site (see Fig. 3). In these circumstances, CEA may be the more prudent choice. Other anatomic CAS exclusionary criteria include thrombus at the treatment site (Fig. 4), long subtotal occlusion (string sign), and, of course, total occlusion.

Calcification at the angioplasty site can be problematic. Calcified plaque resists expansion and if it responds to the angioplasty, it is by fracturing, rather than by stretching or compressing. Expansion of the lumen occurs by stretching of the less

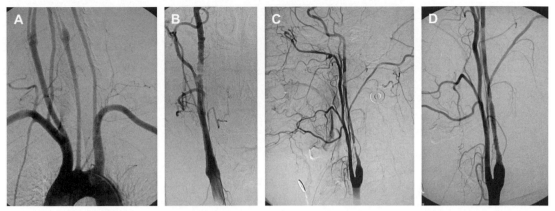

Fig. 1. A 47-year-old woman with left carotid transient ischemic attacks. (*A*) Left anterior oblique arteriogram of the aortic arch, demonstrating a type I arch with a small left internal carotid artery. (*B*) Anteroposterior right common carotid arteriogram, demonstrating irregular, alternating dilation of the right internal carotid artery, which is a diagnostic of fibromuscular hyperplasia. This finding demonstrates the value of examining the opposite carotid artery. (*C*) Lateral left common carotid arteriogram, demonstrating a near occlusion of the internal carotid artery approximately 2 cm above its origin. (*D*) Lateral left common carotid arteriogram after placement of a 6-mm × 20-mm Precise stent. The self-expanding stent dilated the internal carotid artery, so an angioplasty was not necessary.

involved (more normal) carotid wall. The goal of angioplasty when there is heavily calcified plaque at the angioplasty site is a reduction of the stenosis to less than 50%. Even if dilation to a more normal lumen has somehow been achieved with an aggressive angioplasty, this lumen will not be maintained by the stent because of the recoil of the residual artery wall. Attempts at overcoming the resistance of the heavily calcified arterial wall may lead to arterial rupture [3].

During the review of the patient's arteriogram, the status of the opposite carotid artery and any vertebral collaterals is also informative and is particularly important if there are significant stenoses or

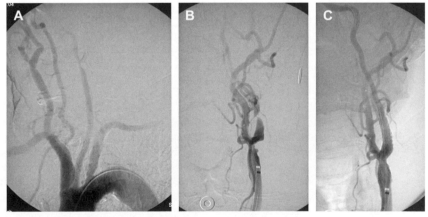

Fig. 2. A 78-year-old man who had bilateral CEAs years previously. He now has left carotid transient ischemic attacks. (*A*) Left anterior oblique arch aortogram, demonstrating heavy calcifications due to atherosclerosis within the aortic arch and a type II–type III origin to the brachiocephalic vessels. Extremely slow flow in the left carotid artery causes it to fill poorly. (*B*) Anteroposterior left common carotid arteriogram after a Simmons 2 catheter was exchanged for a 6F Shuttle sheath, demonstrating severe recurrent atherosclerosis with an ulcerated plaque in the distal left common carotid artery and a very high-grade stenosis in the internal carotid artery, 2 cm beyond its origin. The flow in the internal carotid artery is very slow. (*C*) Anteroposterior left common carotid arteriogram after angioplasty with a 5-mm × 40-mm Savvy balloon and placement of a 10-mm × 40-mm Precise stent across the bifurcation, revealing patency of the internal carotid artery and smoothing of the irregularities in the distal left common carotid artery. The guidewire can be observed across the CAS site with its tip in the petrous carotid artery.

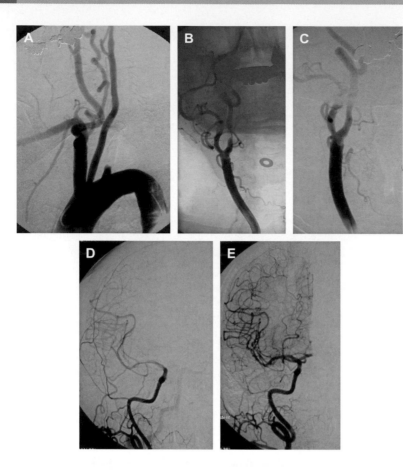

Fig. 3. A 79-year-old woman who had active right carotid distribution transient ischemic attacks and was not a candidate for CEA because of her severe chronic obstructive pulmonary disease, hypertension, and severe peripheral vascular disease. (*A*) Left anterior oblique arch aortogram, demonstrating a type III arch configuration and an occluded left subclavian artery. The right common carotid artery is very tortuous and the right vertebral artery is extremely tortuous. (*B*) Anteroposterior right common carotid arteriogram, demonstrating a high-grade stenosis in the right internal carotid artery, which extends beyond the level of the mandible, increasing the risk for CEA. (*C*) Anteroposterior right common carotid arteriogram after angioplasty with a 4-mm × 40-mm Savvy balloon and placement of an 8-mm × 30-mm Precise stent, demonstrating restoration of a normal lumen. (*D*) Anteroposterior right common carotid arteriogram of the head before the CAS, demonstrating poor filling of the intracranial right carotid distribution because of the internal carotid artery stenosis in the neck. The right anterior cerebral and right posterior cerebral arteries show no filling, and the right middle cerebral artery has unopacified blood mixing with the contrast. (*E*) Anteroposterior right common carotid arteriogram after the CAS, demonstrating filling of the right A1 segment, filling of the right posterior cerebral artery, and now excellent filling of the right middle cerebral artery. Frequently, after angioplasty of high-grade lesions, there is increased flow in the distribution. Because of this, blood pressure must be monitored and controlled tightly.

occlusions and the operator is contemplating using flow reversal with the Parodi anti-embolism system. Although the patient may tolerate cessation or reversal of flow for short periods during the procedure, the risks could be higher than with the filter-type devices.

If the patient's previous evaluation has been with Doppler ultrasound, MR angiography, or CT angiography, a formal arteriogram is performed immediately before the contemplated angioplasty and stenting. In most instances, the arteriogram is performed after placement of a 5F sheath in one of the femoral arteries. The 5F catheters are used for the arch aortography and the selective diagnostic arteriograms, which consist of an aortic arch, bilateral common carotid injections in the neck and head, and at least one vertebral artery (see Fig. 1). Evaluation of the intracranial circulation excludes more significant intracranial stenosis than the target carotid artery. Thus, the appropriateness of the proposed intervention and the suitability of the accompanying vasculature and planned access routes can all be determined before the procedure.

Embolic protection devices

EPDs have been approved recently for use with CAS. The theory behind their design is reasonable because most CVAs and transient ischemic attacks (TIAs) during CAS are caused by emboli. Whether the emboli are due to thrombus formation on the

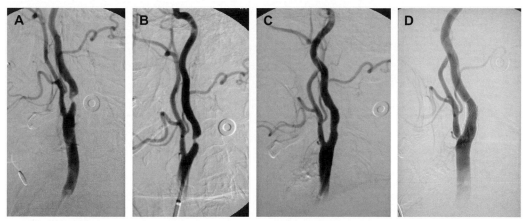

Fig. 4. A 54-year-old woman with a history of a recent right carotid distribution stroke and ongoing transient ischemic attacks despite antiplatelet therapy. She had received radiation therapy for a lymphoma 15 years previously and has had no evidence of recurrence. (*A*) Lateral right common carotid arteriogram in preparation for an angioplasty, demonstrating a high-grade stenosis in the internal carotid artery 1 cm beyond its origin. A filling defect just above the stenosis is a thrombus. (*B*) Lateral right common carotid arteriogram, demonstrating no change in the stenosis after anticoagulation for 1 month, but the thrombus has lysed in the now-asymptomatic patient. (*C*) Lateral right common carotid arteriogram after angioplasty with a 5-mm × 20-mm Savvy balloon and placement of a 9-mm × 30-mm Smart stent across the bifurcation, demonstrating restoration of a normal luminal diameter. (*D*) Lateral right common carotid arteriogram 4 years later, showing persistent patency of the common carotid artery. Slight intimal hyperplasia does not compromise the lumen. The external carotid artery remains patent.

various catheters and devices, platelet aggregation, or liberated atheromatous debris does not matter because the effect is the same, obstruction of the cranial arterial vessels. Only rarely are procedural ischemic events related to hypoperfusion, which is usually due to hypotension and bradycardia. Therefore, the concept of embolic protection is reasonable.

Currently, the four approved EPD systems are all filters with pores that allow blood to pass, but capture emboli or debris. They are mounted on a guidewire, the tip of which must first cross the stenosis; then, the restrained filter crosses the area. This procedure requires a residual lumen of approximately 2 mm. If the lumen is smaller, an unprotected angioplasty with a small balloon must be performed to allow passage of the guidewire and filter. In both instances, risks include obstruction of the lumen, dislodgement of debris (emboli), and dissection. The EPD wires and filters are not as readily maneuverable as standard .014- or .018-in guidewires. Moreover, the filter may not trap all the emboli because of imperfect apposition to the walls of the carotid. It may also become clogged with debris, which significantly obstructs flow. The four FDA-approved EPDs approved by the Food and Drug Administration (FDA) for CAS are available in varying sizes, depending on the size of the artery in which they are to be placed. They should be slightly larger than the internal carotid artery to

assure wall-filter apposition. The first approved EPD was the Accunet, initially developed by Guidant (St. Paul, MN), which has been sold to Abbott (Abbott Park, North Chicago, IL) (Fig. 5). Abbott also has an EPD named the Emboshield. Recently, approval for the Angioguard (Cordis Neurovascular, Miami Lakes, FL) (Fig. 6) and the Spider (eV3, Irvine, CA) has been granted. A similar filter device approved for use in the heart but not for the carotid artery is the FilterWire EZ from Boston Scientific (Fig. 7).

Another not-yet-approved distal EPD is a microballoon, which is placed across the stenosis and inflated. The advantage is complete obstruction to distal embolization. The disadvantages are the resultant complete obstruction to internal carotid artery flow, which is not tolerated in about 5% of patients, and the need to cross the stenosis.

An entirely different concept that is not yet approved for use in the carotid artery is the Parodi anti-embolism system. With this device, the technique is changed; the lesion is not crossed until the EPD is in place (Fig. 8). A large-bore guiding catheter with a balloon at its tip is placed in the common carotid artery. Through the guiding catheter lumen, a second, smaller balloon is positioned in the external carotid. Femoral venous access is also obtained. After the angioplasty device is ready to be positioned, the balloon in the common carotid artery is inflated, thereby obstructing flow.

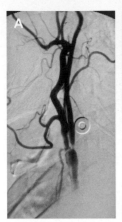
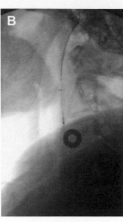
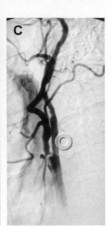

Fig. 5. A 56-year-old woman with a right middle cerebral artery infarction 1 month previously, from which she has recovered. (*A*) Lateral right common carotid arteriogram, demonstrating a high-grade stenosis at the origin of the right internal carotid artery. Because the internal carotid artery is slightly smaller than the external carotid artery, the stenosis, by NASCET criteria, becomes 99%. (*B*) Lateral radiograph of the neck with a 5-mm Accunet EPD deployed in the internal carotid artery. (*C*) Lateral right common carotid arteriogram after angioplasty with a 4-mm × 20-mm Viatrac Plus balloon, and placement of a tapered 7-mm-to-10-mm–diameter × 30-mm–length Acculink stent across the bifurcation, revealing restoration of the normal luminal diameter at the origin of the internal carotid artery. The irregularity in the internal carotid artery above the angioplasty site is due to spasm.

The balloon in the external carotid artery is also inflated. The balloon guide catheter then becomes a conduit for reversed flow from the opposite carotid artery or vertebral basilar system. This flow is directed through a filter and returned to the patient through the femoral vein. A standard angioplasty and stent procedure is then performed. At the conclusion of the CAS procedure, the balloon in the external carotid artery is deflated and removed. The guide catheter balloon is then deflated. The major advantage to this system is that the lesion does not have to be crossed without the protection in place. The major disadvantage is that not all patients have sufficient collateral supply to tolerate the occlusion, and a minor disadvantage is the larger-diameter 10F sheath necessary for insertion of the balloon guide catheter.

The authors have used EPDs for the past year and a half and found that the complication rate is slightly higher because of the learning curve with each EPD.

Although EPDs make intellectual sense, it is unclear whether their use results in a reduction in TIAs, CVAs, and death. Postulated reasons for untoward events despite EPDs include the necessity of crossing the lesion with the filter; movement of the guidewire and filter during the procedure, which may lead to spasm or intimal damage; failure to capture some of the emboli because of incomplete wall apposition; and overwhelming of the filter with debris. Operator inexperience and unfamiliarity with the device may also lead to complications.

Stents

At the time the FDA approved the EPD, they also approved the respective EPD manufacturers' stents.

The self-expanding stents approved for use in the carotid artery are all are constructed of nitinol, which is more conformable than stainless steel, foreshortens minimally, and deploys predictably. The open-cell stents change luminal diameter very quickly and, if properly sized, appose the carotid wall very nicely (Fig. 9). The size of the cell and degree of cell interconnectivity may allow protrusion of atheromatous plaque into the lumen, which is, of course, a disadvantage. In the closed-cell design, each cell buttresses the adjacent cell, which does not accommodate rapid changes in luminal diameter. As a result, the closed-cell stent may not abut the carotid wall completely throughout its length. The strength of this design is that there is less tissue or plaque protrusion after placement, and the cells do not protrude into the lumen to snag EPDs or catheters. Tapering of the stent diameter from distal (smaller) to proximal (larger) is a solution for the size differences between the internal carotid and common carotid arteries. Tapered stents are also available in the open-cell designs (see Fig. 5).

Some closed-cell stents can be resheathed before 75% deployment. The open-cell designs do not permit resheathing. Balloon-mounted stents are used only when they are to be deployed near the carotid origin or high in the internal or external carotid artery, where they are protected by the overlying bony structures. The balloon-mounted stents are very rigid and resist collapse, but when they fail, they do so catastrophically and can only be reopened with another angioplasty, which may require placement of another stent inside the first. The self-expanding stents are not as rigid and are somewhat compressible. They are resilient, which allows re-expansion to their previous diameter.

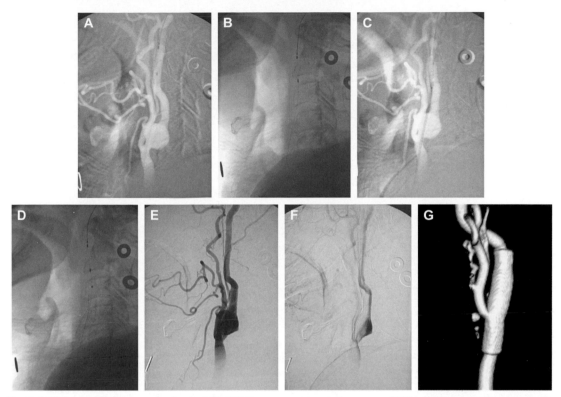

Fig. 6. A 65-year-old woman who had a left CEA 3 years previously because of TIAs due to carotid stenosis. She has had expansion of the internal carotid artery at the CEA site. In an attempt to prevent further expansion, stent placement was undertaken. (*A*) Lateral road-mapped image, demonstrating the dilated proximal left internal carotid artery just beyond its origin. A 7-mm Angioguard has been placed into the internal carotid artery above the site. (*B*) Lateral radiograph more clearly showing the guidewire and the expanded Angioguard. (*C*) Lateral road-mapped image showing positioning of the 7-mm × 40-mm Precise stent across the dilated CEA site and the bifurcation. (*D*) Lateral radiograph, demonstrating the stent bridging the dilated site. The Angioguard remains in place. (*E*) Lateral left common carotid arteriogram after the Angioguard has been collapsed and removed. The stent bridging the internal carotid artery and the dilated section, and in the common carotid artery, is readily apparent. (*F*) Lateral delayed image from the left common carotid arteriogram, demonstrating the slowed flow in the dilated segment. Presumably with time, fibrosis will restore a more normal lumen. The patient remained on aspirin and clopidogrel bisulphate for 3 months to ensure that this was a gradual process. (*G*) Computerized tomographic angiography 3 months poststenting, showing restoration of the normal lumen diameter. The pseudoaneurysm is filled with clot.

Guide catheter selection

The selection of a guide catheter depends on the procedure. If standard angioplasty followed by stent placement is planned, then use of a long guide catheter or sheath is suggested. The size depends on the vessel to be dilated and the devices used. Some of the larger self-expanding stents require 6F or 7F lumen guide catheters. One must be cognizant of the limitations of the guide catheter in placing the devices. The authors have found that the Shuttle (Cook, Inc., Bloomington, IN) provides enough support for the procedure. This sheath is packaged with a removable long-tapered vessel dilator, which enables the sheath to be passed through the soft tissues of the groin and the wall of the femoral artery.

In addition, the tip is well marked, and the lumen on the appropriate-sized sheath adequate for placement of the devices.

Exchange guidewire

Several types of exchange-length wires are available, including the standard heparin-coated steel wires, nitinol wires, and various coated hydrophilic wires. The most useful has a soft, flexible, 2-mm J tip at the end of 60 cm of hydrophilic coating that remains in the carotid artery and aortic arch while the remaining 240 cm of nonhydrophilic wire is in the aorta and outside the patient. The wire is somewhat slick and one must be careful to perform the exchange with fluoroscopy over the neck to assure guidewire

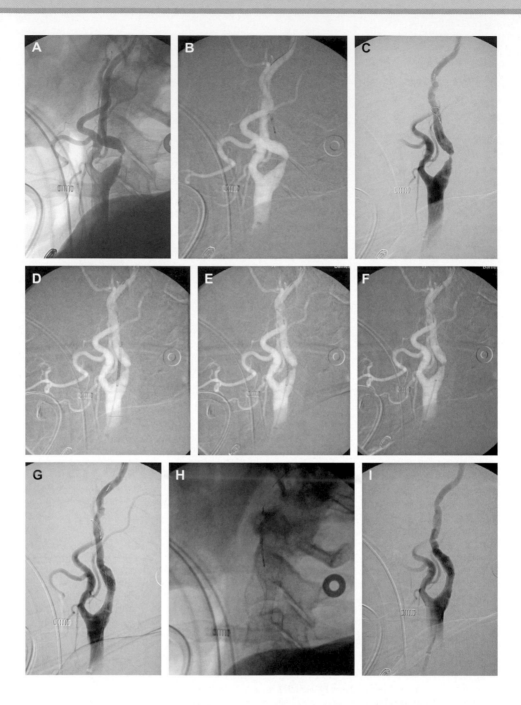

and catheter stability. When the catheter is being withdrawn, the operator may lose control of this slick wire at the groin. A firm grip will prevent this loss of control from happening. The advantage to the J tip of this wire is that it folds upon itself and will not go across a stenosis. Additionally, the last 10 cm of the wire are flexible and radiopaque. If the operator has difficulty controlling the hydrophilic wire, standard 3-mm J-tipped heparin-coated steel wires, which are widely available, may be used.

Guide catheter placement

If the diagnostic arteriogram has been performed before the day of CAS, the femoral artery is accessed with placement of a 5F short sheath and a sample of blood is obtained for activated clotting time for a baseline value. Then the procedure continues as if the diagnostic portion had been performed at the same time. Using one of the diagnostic catheters, the target carotid artery is selected, the guidewire placed, and the target carotid artery catheterized. Then, using an exchange-length guide-wire, first the diagnostic catheter and then the sheath is removed.

The exchange is facilitated by performing a road map arteriogram of the appropriate area of the neck before insertion of the exchange-length wire. The tip of the exchange-length wire is usually placed in the external carotid artery for placement of the guide catheter. If the external carotid artery is stenotic or occluded, the tip of the wire is maintained below the common carotid bifurcation. In this latter instance, the stability of the heparin-coated steel wire may be lacking unless it is very stiff. Substituting a more appropriate guidewire usually allows successful placement of the guide catheter or sheath.

Over the exchange-length guidewire, usually a 6F 80-cm–long Shuttle sheath is placed in the common carotid artery. The tip of the Shuttle sheath, which has a banded marker, is advanced over the obturator when the tip of the latter is in the common carotid artery below the level of stenosis.

Satisfactory placement of the guide catheter is confirmed with a test injection of contrast material. If views of the cranial vasculature have not been obtained, this is done now. Finally, arteriography of the area of stenosis is performed to evaluate the degree of stenosis and the characterization and localization of the plaque, and to obtain a working projection. It is essential that the working projection contain the guide catheter tip, the best view of the route to the stenosis, and the position of the working guidewire.

Medications

After the guide catheter has been placed, the patient is administered intravenous heparin at a dosage of 70 to 100 mg per kg. The activated clotting time is again monitored to assess adequate anticoagulation before crossing the lesion with a guidewire for EPD placement, angioplasty, and stenting. Activated clotting time should be 250 to 300 seconds; if necessary, additional heparin is administered.

Intravenous atropine (0.6–0.8 mg) or glycopyrrolate (0.2–0.4 mg) is administered intravenously for prophylaxis of bradycardia and hypotension in patients who have not undergone prior CEA.

Contrast material is injected and biplane road maps are obtained. The authors feel that the road maps are of higher fidelity than the fluorofade on their angiographic equipment. Any patient movement means the road maps must be repeated to ensure accuracy of the registration for the procedure.

Over-the-wire devices

The operator has some choice in the devices used in CAS. Initially, balloons and stents were only available for over-the-wire use. The disadvantage of over-the-wire systems is the requisite use of the 300-cm wire, which requires two operators. The advantage, though, is the greater stability of the wire tip due to less movement and the slightly greater shaft size.

Rapid exchange

Following developments in cardiology, rapid exchange devices have become available for CAS. These devices require a .014-in guidewire, which passes through the tip of the angioplasty catheter or stent delivery device and then exits the catheter approximately 25 cm from the tip (see **Figs. 5 and 7**). With these devices, a single operator can hold the wire in position and advance the various catheters over it. Similarly, holding the guidewire in position, the single operator can withdraw the

---

Fig. 7. A 74-year-old man receiving coumadin for atrial fibrillation had three episodes of severe epistaxis requiring nasal packing. The last episode was so severe that angiography and embolization were requested. A diagnostic left common carotid arteriogram demonstrated a severe stenosis in the left internal carotid artery with retrograde flow in the left ophthalmic artery, which precluded embolization of the left internal maxillary artery. The high-grade stenosis in the left internal carotid artery was neurologically asymptomatic. (*A*) Lateral left common carotid arteriogram, demonstrating the tip of the 6F guide catheter in the left common carotid artery below the bifurcation. (*B*) Lateral road-mapped image with the EPD and its delivery catheter crossed the stenosis into the internal carotid artery. The EPD has not been deployed. (*C*) Lateral left common carotid arteriogram demonstrating the expansion of the EPD in a straight segment of the internal carotid artery above the stenosis. Note that the contrast passes through the EPD into the internal carotid artery above. (*D*) Lateral road-mapped image during placement of the self-expanding stent across the stenosis. Note how the stent has distorted the internal carotid artery so that it appears to be outside the vessel lumen. (*E*) Lateral road-mapped image during expansion of the stent across the stenosis. (*F*) Lateral road-mapped image after complete expansion of the stent. (*G*) Lateral left common carotid arteriogram after the CAS has been performed, restoring a near-normal lumen. The EPD remains in place. (*H*) Native lateral view of the neck, with the capturing catheter in place collapsing the EPD. (*I*) Lateral left common carotid arteriogram after the EPD has been removed, demonstrating slight irregularity due to spasm at the site of the EPD, but wide patency of the internal carotid artery.

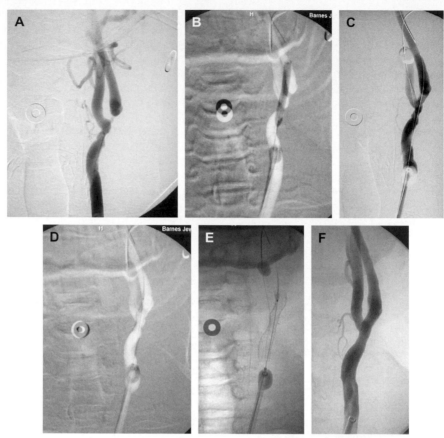

Fig. 8. A 63-year-old man who had a left CEA 18 months previously for amaurosis fugax and is currently asymptomatic. (*A*) Anteroposterior left common carotid arteriogram, revealing a 95% stenosis at the origin of the internal carotid artery and a 50% stenosis of the distal left common carotid artery. Crossing this with a filter-type EPD was thought to be dangerous, so the Parodi anti-embolism system was used "off-label." (*B*) Anteroposterior road-mapped image, demonstrating the guide balloon catheter in place, with the guide balloon inflated. Through the guide catheter, a second balloon has been placed into the external carotid artery and inflated. The distended 5-mm × 40-mm Savvy angioplasty balloon across the high-grade stenosis in the proximal internal carotid artery and the guidewire for the angioplasty balloon can be identified. (*C*) Anteroposterior left common carotid arteriography after the angioplasty, demonstrating significant dilation at the angioplasty site. The guidewire across the stenosis, the inflated balloons of the Parodi anti-embolism system in the external carotid artery, and the common carotid artery all can be identified. (*D*) Frontal view from a road-mapped image, demonstrating an 8-mm × 40-mm Precise stent across the angioplasty site in the internal carotid artery and more proximally into the common carotid artery. (*E*) Frontal radiograph, clearly showing the guidewire and the stent across the angioplasty site. The external carotid and common carotid artery balloons contain contrast. (*F*) Anteroposterior left common carotid arteriogram after the balloons have been deflated and withdrawn. The guidewire has also been withdrawn. This arteriogram demonstrates mild irregularity at the angioplasty site but wide patency of the common carotid and internal carotid arteries. Although the lumen is not dilated completely, one must remember that the self-expanding stent exerts some external expansile forces. If this result was not satisfactory, a further angioplasty through the stent with a larger balloon could be performed.

angioplasty catheter or stent delivery device while leaving the wire in place. The major disadvantage is the reduction in the maneuverability of the guidewire in the rapid-exchange design. Another disadvantage seems to be that the .014 wire is very flexible, which decreases stability. Overall, in the authors' experience, there seems to be more motion of the guidewire tip and EPD with rapid-exchange devices.

Order of procedures

Performing endovascular procedures for carotid atherosclerosis has two schools of thought. One recommends that a definitive angioplasty be performed and the stent placed. The other recommends that an initial angioplasty with a relatively small balloon (3- to 4-mm diameter) be performed, the stent placed, and then definitive angioplasty

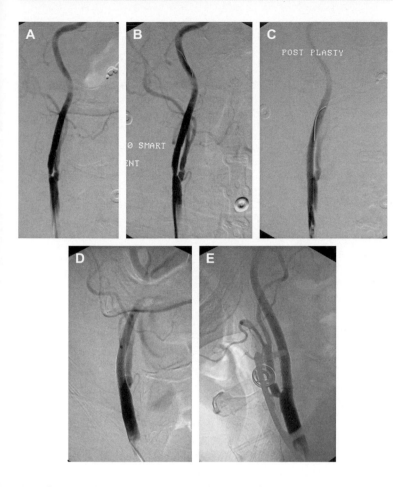

Fig. 9. A 74-year-old man who had undergone bilateral CEAs 5 years previously. He is currently asymptomatic but had a right carotid stenosis on Doppler sonography. (*A*) Anteroposterior right common carotid arteriography, demonstrating a high-grade stenosis at the origin of his internal carotid artery. An angioplasty with a 4-mm × 20-mm Savvy balloon was performed. (*B*) Frontal right common carotid arteriogram after placement of a 9-mm × 30-mm Smart stent across the bifurcation, demonstrating 50% residual stenosis at the origin of the internal carotid artery. (*C*) Frontal right common carotid arteriogram after repeat angioplasty with a 7-mm × 20-mm Opta balloon, revealing satisfactory dilation of the residual stenosis. (*D*) Frontal right common carotid arteriogram 4 years later, revealing ongoing patency of the right internal, external, and common carotid arteries. (*E*) Lateral right common carotid arteriogram, demonstrating patency of all of the vessels and the advantage of the open-cell designed stent, which changes luminal diameters from the internal carotid artery to the common carotid artery relatively quickly.

performed immediately to achieve the final desired size (see Fig. 9). The self-expanding stents exert outward force if appropriately sized and may expand the lumen over the next month after deployment, which should be kept in mind before repeat angioplasty after stent expansion if residual stenosis is 25% to 50% (see Fig. 8). The initial definitive angioplasty proponents believe that it is the angioplasty that releases material from the plaque and therefore they would prefer to perform only one angioplasty. The proponents of the initial angioplasty/stent-placement–definitive angioplasty procedure believe that the stent provides some protection from the release of the atherosclerotic debris when the definitive angioplasty is performed. The counter-argument is that the atherosclerotic material will be forced through the stent when the definitive angioplasty is performed. When an EPD is used, this latter argument is theoretically moot for the multiple angioplasties. However, when a filter-type EPD is used with a residual lumen less than

2 mm, an unprotected angioplasty with a small balloon is necessary to allow passage of the guidewire and filter. Both are then advanced through the recent angioplasty site, which may increase the risk of emboli or dissection. Dissection can be managed by stent placement if the position of a guidewire across the angioplasty site is maintained.

Nonprotected carotid angioplasty and stenting

If the definitive angioplasty route is chosen, the authors use a noncompliant balloon that would reach, at most, a normal luminal diameter, and do not oversize. In a heavily calcified lesion, undersizing is appropriate. One must remember that most of the dilation occurs in the more normal aspects of the vessel, rather than in the plaque. For very short lesions, the authors choose a 2-cm–length balloon and for most other lesions a 4-cm–length balloon. The 4-cm length prevents the

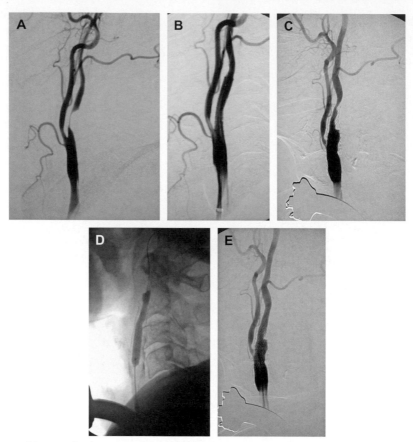

Fig. 10. A 56-year-old man who has received prior radiation therapy and surgery for a laryngeal carcinoma and has left amaurosis fugax. (*A*) Lateral left common carotid arteriogram, demonstrating the internal carotid artery to be threadlike. (*B*) Lateral left common carotid arteriogram after an angioplasty with a 5-mm × 40-mm Savvy balloon and placement of a 9-mm × 40-mm Smart stent with the guidewire in place, demonstrating resolution of the stenosis and ongoing patency of the external carotid artery. (*C*) Lateral left common carotid arteriogram 4 years later, demonstrating intimal hyperplasia narrowing the internal carotid artery and the patent left external carotid artery. The patient remained asymptomatic. (*D*). Lateral radiograph with a 5-mm × 40-mm Savvy balloon in the stent and inflated. An EPD was not used because the stenosis was thought to be due to intimal hyperplasia. (*E*) Lateral left common carotid arteriogram after the angioplasty, demonstrating restoration of a normal luminal diameter of the internal carotid artery. Patients receiving radiation therapy have had nearly all of the recurrent stenoses (16%).

balloon from migrating either proximally or distally as it distends. With a shorter balloon, migration may necessitate several dilations.

To opacify the angioplasty balloon, a mixture of dilute contrast and saline (two thirds contrast, one third saline) is used (see Fig. 8; Fig. 10). Some agents are inappropriate Visipaque because of their viscosity. Using a long, blunt needle, the port for the balloon adapter is flushed with the contrast/saline mixture. A three-way stopcock is attached. On one port, a 10-mL syringe containing the contrast mixture is placed. On the other, the inflation device containing the contrast mixture is attached. After debubbling the two syringes and the three-way stopcock, negative pressure is applied to the 10-mL syringe and then relieved by changing the stopcock

position to allow the contrast from the inflation device to travel to the balloon. This procedure is repeated several times in an effort to remove as much as possible of the air in the dead space. If necessary, the three-way stopcock is removed, the bubbles are flushed from the balloon, and then the three-way stopcock is reattached. The negative pressurization procedure is then repeated so that all the visible bubbles have been removed. The danger of a ruptured balloon is compounded by gas bubbles in the system. Although the operator cannot predict balloon failure, adhering to the recommended inflation pressures, staying below the rated burst pressure, and eliminating all the possible gas bubbles will lessen the impact of this type of failure.

Angioplasty

After the guidewire has been inserted through the balloon, its tip is shaped into a gentle J and withdrawn to the tip of the balloon. The angioplasty catheter and wire are inserted through the rotating hemostatic valve into the guide catheter. The tip of the guidewire is advanced as the balloon emerges from the guide catheter into the common carotid artery. Guidance is provided by fluoroscopy and the road-mapped image. The tip of the guidewire is manipulated across the stenosis using the torque device.

The balloon is positioned so that the central portion is in the area of greatest stenosis (see **Figs. 7 and 10**). The balloon is expanded slowly over minutes to its nominal diameter at its nominal pressure. The burst pressure is usually several atmospheres higher than the nominal pressure. One must remember that the rated burst pressure is two standard deviations below the pressure at which most balloons burst, which provides an element of safety.

After the angioplasty balloon has been collapsed, it can be withdrawn, leaving the guidewire across the angioplasty site. Again, this procedure is performed under fluoroscopy.

Stent placement

The diameter of the stent should be 1 to 2 mm larger than the largest-diameter vessel in which it is to be deployed. Oversizing the stent has little downside, but undersizing creates dead space between the stent and the carotid wall, which probably increases the risk of thromboembolism and may lead to myointimal hyperplasia. The selected stent is positioned using the initial road map or, if there is movement, a new road map image, so that it covers the lesion (see **Fig. 7**). The authors believe that attempting to size stents precisely to the length of the lesion and then attempting to position the stent precisely to this length leads to the placement of multiple stents. This result is usually because of inherent forward motion in the self-expanding stent, so that the distal normal portion of the carotid artery has more stent than desired, which leaves the more proximal portion uncovered. If the lesion is not covered by the deployed stent, the stent delivery catheter must be removed (leaving the guidewire in place) and a second stent positioned so that it overlaps the first by approximately 25%. This additional stent must be at least the same diameter as the first, or 1 mm larger, so that it can be applied as close as possible to the initial stent wall. At times, the positioning of the additional stent may be difficult because the stiff tip of the delivery device brushes against the deployed stent. The struts of the deployed stent become obstacles to the positioning of the next stent. Sometimes, turning the patient's head or elevating the chin will change the orientation of the wire and catheter within the stent, permitting positioning of the second stent. The authors recommend placing a longer stent initially, so the degree of precision in its placement does not need to be so great. Frequently, placing a longer stent results in the stent being placed across the carotid bifurcation. In their experience, placing the stent across the external carotid artery does not affect its patency. After stent deployment, the delivery catheter is withdrawn under fluoroscopy; the wire is left across the CAS site.

When the initial angioplasty/stent placement–definitive angioplasty procedure is chosen, the stent delivery catheter must be removed and the larger (definitive) angioplasty balloon positioned (see **Fig. 9**). This angioplasty is similar to the other angioplasties; however, it is performed within the stent using fluoroscopy for guidance.

Carotid angioplasty and stenting using embolic protection devices

CAS with the EPD adds the step of placing the guidewire-mounted filter across the stenosis, similar to crossing the stenosis with the guidewire for the angioplasty balloon in the initial step of the nonprotected CAS procedure. After the filter is across the stenosis and deployed, its delivery catheter is removed, leaving the guidewire across the lesion (see **Figs. 5 and 7**). The filter-bearing guidewire will serve as guidance for the subsequent rapid-exchange–system angioplasty balloon and the stenting procedure, which are exactly the same for nonprotected and protected CAS procedures. After removal of the stent delivery device, the filters are retrieved by being collapsed with a capturing or retraction catheter. If large amounts of debris are captured, the filter may not collapse completely and must be retracted through the deployed stent, on which they can snag. Usually, advancing the filter wire and then the guide catheter to near the snag site will free the filter and allow retraction into the guide catheter. Obviously, manipulation should be kept to a minimum at the angioplasty and stenting site. Access across the angioplasty and stenting site is lost with filter-wire retrieval.

Prior to withdrawal of the guidewire in nonprotected procedures and before filter retrieval in EPD-assisted procedures, angiography is repeated to evaluate the adequacy of the CAS procedure and any possible thrombus development (see **Fig. 7**). The intracranial circulation is evaluated to assess the flow dynamics, the possibility of embolic phenomena, or any distal carotid injury or spasm (see **Figs. 3 and 5**). Thrombus development at the angioplasty and stenting site is usually due to platelet aggregation and may be treated with 2 to 10 mg of intra-arterial IIb/IIIa inhibitors in 2-mg aliquots with a microcatheter at the site. For intracranial thrombus, microcatheterization of the affected vessel is necessary, particularly with flow-limiting lesions. Similar amounts of IIb/IIIa inhibitor can be administered as in the common carotid or internal carotid arteries. Pursuit of thrombus into the smaller intracranial vessels is dangerous and should be avoided. Thrombolytics, such as urokinase or tissue plasminogen activators, have also been used. Because premedication with antiplatelet agents has become standard preoperative care, thrombus formation is now rare. Absence of response to the IIb/IIIA inhibitors and the lytics suggests that the filling defect is due to atheroma rather than thrombus. Only medical therapy may be effective in this latter instance. Vasospasm may be observed and resolve spontaneously. Severe, nonresolving spasm may be treated with 10 mg of verapamil in 10 mL of saline over 10 minutes infused intra-arterially near the site. Similarly, nitroglycerin, 200 to 400 μg, can be administered intra-arterially to relieve vasospasm.

The guide catheter is withdrawn. If use of a closure device is contemplated, arteriography of the iliofemoral arterial system is performed. If the vessel is suitable, hemostasis can be obtained.

If a decision is made to remove the sheath later that day, the long sheath is exchanged for a similar-sized short sheath and sutured in position. A sterile dressing is applied. The catheter is slowly perfused with heparinized saline (2000 units in 1000 mL) under arterial pressure at a keep-open rate.

The activated clotting time is monitored again to be certain that it is not too high. Usually, additional heparin is not administered again.

Medical therapy of complications

Vasovagal reactions usually are transient and respond to fluids and repeat doses of atropine or glycopyrrolate. If the hypotension does not resolve, intravenous phenylephrine, 10 to 100 mg/min, or dopamine, 5 to 15 μg/kg/min, should be available. If the bradycardia does not resolve, external, or even temporary, transvenous pacemaking may be necessary. Hypertension is to be avoided, and systolic blood pressure that rises above 180 mm Hg should be treated with labetalol, 20-mg intravenous bolus over 2 minutes, or a 0.5 to 2 mg/min intravenous infusion.

Postprocedural care

The patient is observed in the intensive care unit overnight. Close attention is paid to the neurologic status, and blood pressure is monitored closely and treated if necessary. If the patient is unchanged the following morning, is able to eat, void, and ambulate, he/she is discharged to home. Activity is increased gradually, so that at 2 weeks, an office worker could return to work and at 4 weeks, a manual laborer could return to work. The patient is maintained on aspirin and clopidogrel bisulphate for 30 days after the procedure and then 325 mg aspirin indefinitely. Baseline Doppler studies are

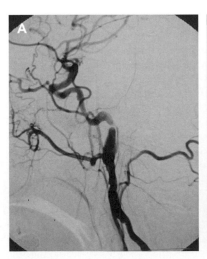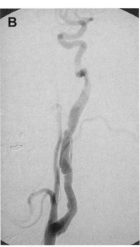

Fig. 11. A 42-year-old man with left carotid TIAs after "popping" his neck. (*A*) Lateral left common carotid arteriogram, demonstrating marked irregularity in the internal carotid artery extending to the level of the skull base, a dissection with a large pseudoaneurysm. Only a thin residual lumen can be observed posterior to the pseudoaneurysm just below the skull base. This lumen was traversed with a guidewire and a 7-mm × 40-mm Precise stent placed. (*B*) Lateral left common carotid arteriogram 1 year later, demonstrating residual irregularity in the internal carotid artery from its origin to the skull base, but no residual stenosis. The wind sock deformity of the pseudoaneurysm has been obliterated by the stent.

usually obtained at 6 months, and then at yearly intervals.

Other indications for carotid angioplasty and stenting (dissection)

Dissection of the carotid artery, an important cause of CVA in young patients, may be spontaneous, traumatic, or iatrogenic (**Fig. 11**). Medical or surgical therapies have not been evaluated definitively with controlled trials. If neurologic symptoms develop or progress despite medical therapy (usually antiplatelet or anticoagulant agents), they are thought to be due to thromboemboli, which may arise from either the stenosis at the dissection site or the development of a pseudoaneurysm with a narrow neck, resulting in stasis within the sac, or a combination of both. The authors have treated 26 patients with dissections; 54% were neurologically symptomatic [4]. The cause was spontaneous in eight, traumatic in nine, and iatrogenic in nine. The traumatic or spontaneous dissections occurred at, or near, the skull base in 77%, whereas the iatrogenic dissections occurred near the common carotid bifurcation in 89%. The procedures were performed without EPDs, which were not available for this application. Because most patients will have been treated conservatively for a while, identification of the true lumen usually is not problematic. The channel that leads back into the lumen above the dissection is chosen for stenting, the guidewire manipulated to traverse the area, and the stent deployed. The goal of the treatment is the same as for atherosclerotic narrowing, restoration of the normal lumen. Usually, placing a self-expanding stent restores the stenotic lumen, making angioplasty superfluous. Only rarely will an accompanying pseudoaneurysm not be compressed by the stent. Usually, the iatrogenic pseudoaneurysm requires coil embolization through the stent struts because of the initial presentation of bleeding from the pseudoaneurysm.

In the authors' patients who had dissection-related stenosis, all but one had restoration of a normal lumen. The one who did not had only a residual 50% stenosis. The TIA rate after stenting was 10%, which would suggest EPDs (which were not used) may be of value, despite angiographic absence of thrombus at the dissection site. No CVAs occurred. In two patients, the treated carotid artery was occluded (one patient at 1 month and the other at 3 months), but no anticoagulation or antiplatelet agents were administered in one patient and the other only received aspirin.

Overall, stenting of carotid dissections is a logical extension of carotid therapy, with relatively low risk of complications.

Carotid angioplasty and stenting results

In the authors' experience with symptomatic and asymptomatic patients, CAS without EPD has been reasonably safe in more than 250 procedures. Their opinions have been shaped over the last 10 years by treating patients who would be excluded by the NASCET study criteria. During those 10 years, if the patient was a good operative candidate for CEA, that procedure was performed. Analysis of the results of CAS in different groups of patients supports the authors' opinion that the procedure is reasonably safe, results in persistent restoration of a normal lumen, and reduces the subsequent incidence of CVA and TIA.

In the authors' group of 167 CAS-treated patients without EPDs, the procedural CVA rate was 2.4% and the TIA rate, 3.6% [5]. The 30-day composite postprocedural stroke and death rate was 5%. Prior ischemic symptoms were associated strongly with intraprocedural thromboembolic events.

Radiation-associated atherosclerotic stenosis is a high-risk factor for CEA and was excluded from NASCET entry criteria because most of the patients would have had neck dissections before the radiation therapy, both of which obscure tissue planes. In the authors' 23 CAS procedures performed after radiation therapy, the CVA rate was 4% without TIAs occurring. Recurrences of significant stenosis required 16% of treated vessels to be retreated (see **Figs. 4 and 10**) [6].

Elderly people (79 years of age or older) currently are being excluded from CREST and have been recommended not to undergo CAS [7]. The authors' group of 20 elderly patients who underwent CAS included no strokes and only one TIA. Mean follow-up of 2 years demonstrated no new strokes in these patients (CJ Moran, DT Cross, CP Derdeyn, unpublished data, 2007) (see **Fig. 3**).

Another group of patients were excluded from NASCET because they had a prior CEA, which was thought to place them at higher risk for local and neurologic complications [8]. In the authors' group of 75 patients who had CEA, the procedural CVA rate was 3.6% and the TIA rate, 2.4%. The composite 30-day CVA, myocardial infarction, and death rate was 6%. The recurrent stenosis was reduced from a mean of 81% to no significant stenosis (see **Figs. 2, 6, 8, and 9**) [9].

The authors' experience supporting CAS for carotid disease is corroborated in some reports. A review of the literature through 2002 found that the risk of CVA and death was 5.5% without EPDs in those patients undergoing CAS [10]. Most recently, CAS was evaluated by registries conducted for CE marking approval in Europe and investigational device exemption to acquire FDA premarket approval in the United States. These registries surveyed patients considered at high risk for CEA, but did not include control groups. The ARCHeR study found a 30-day myocardial infarction, CVA, death rate of 8.3% for CAS [11]. The BEACH study found a myocardial infarction, CVA, death rate of 5.8% [12]. A study of the CREATE trial found a 30-day myocardial infarction, CVA, death rate of 6.2% [13].

Recent randomized clinical trials have compared CAS with EPD to CEA. The SAPPHIRE trial was stopped prematurely because of slow enrollment and because many patients were considered too high a risk for CEA. However, in a total of 334 nonrandomized patients in that study, the 30-day incidence of myocardial infarction, CVA, death was 4.8% after CAS and 9.8% after CEA [14]. A meta-analysis of five randomized clinical trials comparing CAS to CEA found no difference in myocardial infarction, CVA, death at 30 days between the two procedures (8.1% versus 7.8%) [15].

However, recently (late 2006), two trials have suggested that CAS may not be equal to CEA. In a trial (SPACE) in which EPD use was at the discretion of the interventionalist, CAS was inferior to CEA [16]. The second study (EVA-3S) was a French study (using five different stents and seven different EPDs) that found CAS with mandated EPD had a CVA/death rate of 9.6%, compared with only 3.9% for CEA [17]. The CAS showed no difference, with or without EPD. The major criticism of this trial has been the lack of experience of the investigators and operators [18].

Summary

Notwithstanding the results of the various trials, and with FDA approval for EPDs and accompanying stents, the equation has yet another factor, reimbursement for CAS. According to one study, the cost of CAS and CEA show little difference [19]. The Centers for Medicare and Medicaid Services (CMS) at first issued national coverage determination for CAS for patients who are at high risk for CEA with a symptomatic stenosis greater than or equal to 70% and who are less than 80 years old. This agency then proposed on February 1, 2007, to extend coverage only to those at high risk for CEA and who have an asymptomatic stenosis greater than or equal to 80%. Furthermore, CAS is covered only when an EPD is used, even if deployment of the EPD is not technically possible. CMS comment that if deployment of the distal EPD is not possible, the procedure should be aborted, given the risks of CAS without distal embolic protection.

This decision would seem to ignore the lessons from NASCET, which demonstrated that CVA risks for these patients at 2 years with medical therapy

is 26%, which is much higher than that for unprotected angioplasty [20]. The practitioner must balance the risks and benefits of CAS, CEA, and medical therapy for patients who have carotid disease, regardless of the standards of third-party payors.

Overall, the procedure of angioplasty and stenting is similar to many other interventional techniques. If the practitioner is diligent in applying excellent angiographic techniques, is cognizant of the pitfalls, performs the procedure in a repeatable, reproducible manner, selects patients appropriately, and administers antiplatelet agents, the results should be worthwhile.

References

[1] Morgenstern LB, Fox AJ, Sharpe BL, et al. The risks and benefits of carotid endarterectomy in patients with near occlusion of the carotid artery. Neurology 1997;48(4):911–5.

[2] Wholey MH, Wholey MH, Eles G, et al. Evaluation of glycoprotein IIb/IIIa inhibitors in carotid angioplasty and stenting. J Endovasc Ther 2003; 10(1):33–41.

[3] Broadbent LP, Moran CJ, Cross DT III, et al. Management of ruptures complicating angioplasty and stenting of supraaortic arteries: report of two cases and a review of the literature. AJNR Am J Neuroradiol 2003;24(10):2057–61.

[4] Kadkhodayan Y, Jeck DT, Moran CJ, et al. Angioplasty and stenting in carotid dissection with or without associated pseudoaneurysm. AJNR Am J Neuroradiol 2005;26(9):2328–35.

[5] Kadkhodayan Y, Derdeyn CP, Cross DT III, et al. Procedural complications of carotid angioplasty and stent placement without cerebral protection devices. Neurosurg Focus 2005;18(1):E1–7.

[6] Harrod-Kim P, Kadkhodayan Y, Derdeyn CP, et al. Outcomes of carotid angioplasty and stenting for radiation-associated stenosis. AJNR Am J Neuroradiol 2005;26(17):1781–8.

[7] Hobson RW, Howard VJ, Roubin GS, et al. Carotid artery stenting is associated with increased complications in octogenarians: 30-day stroke and death rates in the CREST lead-in phase. J Vasc Surg 2004;40(6):1106–11.

[8] Bond R, Rerkasem K, Rothwell PM. Systematic review of the risks of carotid endarterectomy in relation to the clinical indication for and timing of surgery. Stroke 2003;34(9):2290–303.

[9] Kadkhodayan Y, Moran CJ, Derdeyn CP, et al. Carotid angioplasty and stent placement for restenosis after endarterectomy. Neuroradiology 2007;49(4):357–64.

[10] Kastrup A, Gröschel K, Krapf H, et al. Early outcome of carotid angioplasty and stenting with and without cerebral protection devices; a systematic review of the literature. Stroke 2003;34(3):813–9.

[11] Gray WA, Hopkins LN, Yadav S, et al. Protected carotid stenting in high-surgical-risk patients:

the ARCHeR results. J Vasc Surg 2006;44(2): 258–69.

[12] White CJ, Iyer SS, Hopkins LN, et al. for the BEACH Trial Investigators. Carotid stenting with distal protection in high surgical risk patients: the BEACH trial 30 day results. Catheter Cardiovasc Interv 2006;67(4):503–12.

[13] Safian RD, Bresnahan JF, Jaff MR, et al. Protected carotid stenting in high-risk patients with severe carotid artery stenosis. J Am Coll Cardiol 2006; 47(12):2384–9.

[14] Yadav JS, Wholey MH, Kuntz RE, et al. Protected carotid-artery stenting versus endarterectomy in high-risk patients. N Engl J Med 2004;351(15): 1493–501.

[15] Coward LJ, Featherstone RL, Brown MM. Safety and efficacy of endovascular treatment of carotid artery stenosis compared with carotid endarterectomy; a Cochrane systematic review of the randomized evidence. Stroke 2005;36(4): 905–11.

[16] The SPACE Collaborative Group. 30 day results from the SPACE trial of stent-protected angioplasty versus carotid endarterectomy in symptomatic patients: a randomized non-inferiority trial. Lancet 2006;368(9543):1239–47.

[17] Mas J-L, Chatellier G, Beyssen B, et al. Endarterectomy versus stenting in patients with symptomatic severe carotid stenosis. N Engl JMed 2006;355(16):1660–71.

[18] Furlan AJ. Carotid-artery stenting—case open or closed? N Engl J Med 2006;355(16):1726–9.

[19] Ecker RD, Brown RD Jr, Nichols DA, et al. Cost of treating high-risk symptomatic carotid artery stenosis: stent insertion and angioplasty compared with endarterectomy. J Neurosurg 2004; 101(6):904–7.

[20] North American Symptomatic Carotid Endarterectomy Trial Collaborators. Beneficial effect of carotid endarterectomy in symptomatic patients with high-grade carotid stenosis. N Engl J Med 1991;325(7):445–53.

ELSEVIER
SAUNDERS

NEUROIMAGING
CLINICS
OF NORTH AMERICA

Neuroimag Clin N Am 17 (2007) 355–363

Angioplasty and Stenting for Atherosclerotic Intracranial Stenosis: Rationale for a Randomized Clinical Trial

Colin P. Derdeyn, MD[a],*, Marc I. Chimowitz, MBChB[b]

Atherosclerotic stenosis affecting the major intracranial arterial is a common cause of stroke in North America, particularly in some minority populations [1–3]. Patients presenting with transient ischemic attack (TIA) or stroke and severe (>70% diameter reduction) stenosis are at a very high risk for future stroke [4]. The mechanism of stroke in these patients may be related to thromboembolism resulting from biologic plaque factors, hemodynamic factors resulting from flow reduction beyond the stenosis, or synergistic effects of the two [5,6]. Angioplasty and stenting offer the potential to address both mechanisms and to reduce stroke risk substantially. Angioplasty and stent technology has improved dramatically during recent years.

There are accumulating data on the technical success and safety of these procedures, but the long-term reduction of the risk of stroke remains undetermined. At present, only one device, the Wingspan self-expanding stent (Boston Scientific, Natick, MA), is approved by the Food and Drug Administration (FDA) for use in patients who have symptomatic atherosclerotic stenosis (50%–99%) of intracranial arteries.

This article discusses the outcome of medically treated patients who have intracranial stenosis, drawing heavily from the recently reported Warfarin versus Aspirin for Symptomatic Intracranial Disease (WASID) study [4,7,8]. It then reviews the published data for intracranial angioplasty, with

Support for this work was provided by National Institute of Neurological Disorders and Stroke grants R01 NS051631, R01 NS036643, K24 NS050307, R01 NS051688.
[a] Mallinckrodt Institute of Radiology, Washington University School of Medicine, 510 South Kingshighway Blvd, St. Louis, MO 63110, USA
[b] Emory University School of Medicine, Emory Stroke Program, 1365 Clifton Road NE, Room A4302, Atlanta, GA 30422, USA
* Corresponding author.
E-mail address: derdeync@wustl.edu (C.P. Derdeyn).

neuroimaging.theclinics.com

doi:10.1016/j.nic.2007.05.001

and without stenting. Finally, it discusses the rationale for a randomized trial of angioplasty and stenting for symptomatic intracranial atherosclerotic stenosis.

Epidemiology

Atherosclerotic stenosis of large intracranial arteries accounts for approximately 10% of ischemic strokes that occur in North America. There is racial and ethnic variance in this disease. Intracranial arterial stenosis is responsible for 6% to 10% of ischemic strokes in whites, 6% to 29% of ischemic strokes in blacks, 11% of ischemic strokes in Hispanics, and 22% to 26% of ischemic strokes in Asians [1–3,9]. These figures project to approximately 70,000 strokes per year in the United States [10], compared with the 140,000 strokes caused by extracranial carotid stenosis and 70,000 strokes caused by nonvalvular atrial fibrillation [11,12].

Pathophysiology

The mechanisms of ischemic stroke related to intracranial atherosclerotic disease include thromboembolic factors, such as in situ thrombosis and distal embolism and hemodynamic factors resulting from flow reduction and lack of adequate sources of collateral flow [13–15]. As discussed in the article by Derdeyn in this issue, both mechanisms are commonly involved in most patients and probably are synergistic. Lee and colleagues [15], reviewed diffusion-weighted MR imaging in 63 acute patients who had ischemic stroke and who had stroke who had ipsilateral middle cerebral artery (MCA) disease, 32 of whom showed multiple lesions. Most patients had perforating artery infarcts, either solitary or accompanied by pial or border-zone territory infarcts. These data suggest that local branch occlusion and simultaneous distal embolization is a common stroke mechanism in patients who have MCA disease. The present authors measured hemodynamics in 10 patients who had symptomatic MCA occlusion or stenosis, using positron-emission tomography [13]. Blood flow and oxygen extraction were normal in four of the five patients who had stenosis. These data suggest that most patients who have symptomatic intracranial stenosis are symptomatic as the result of thromboembolic factors.

Nevertheless, hemodynamic impairment is a risk factor for stroke in patients who have intracranial occlusive disease, just it is as in those who have extracranial carotid artery occlusive disease. Amin-Hanjani and colleagues [16] measured quantitative bulk flow in the basilar artery and its branches in 50 patients who had symptomatic vertebrobasilar disease. Forty-seven of the 50 patients were followed for a mean of 28 months, although those who had low flow were offered intervention. None of the 31 patients who had normal distal flow had a recurrent event. Several of the 16 patients who had low flow suffered recurrent strokes before intervention.

Outcome of medically treated patients

The WASID trial generated the best estimates of the outcome of medically treated patients who have symptomatic intracranial atherosclerotic disease [4,7,8]. This section reviews the data from this study in detail, including secondary analyses identifying particularly high-risk patients. It also reviews the current data for risk factor management in this population. These data are important, because angioplasty and stenting should target the patients at the highest risk for stroke with medical therapy. Most of these patients have vascular risk factors that should be treated as well.

Warfarin versus Aspirin for Symptomatic Intracranial Disease trial

The WASID trial was a randomized, double-blinded, multicenter, controlled study designed to determine the relative efficacy of aspirin (1300 mg/d by mouth) versus anticoagulation with warfarin (target international normalized ratio [INR], 2.0–3.0) in patients who had angiographically proven 50% to 99% stenosis of a major intracranial artery and a recent TIA or minor stroke [4].

At total of 569 patients were enrolled between 1999 and 2003. The median time from qualifying event to randomization was 17 days. Mean follow-up was 1.8 years. Baseline clinical characteristics between the two groups were similar. These baseline characteristics also were very similar to those in prior clinical trials in patients who had atherosclerotic extracranial carotid stenosis or occlusion [5,17,18]. The majority of patients had a history of hypertension or smoking. A large minority had diabetes or a prior coronary artery disease. Subjects could be screened by transcranial Doppler, magnetic resonance angiography, or CT angiography. Enrollment required confirmation of 50% to 99% stenosis with catheter angiography [19]. The study drug was discontinued by more warfarin patients than aspirin patients (28.4% versus 16.4%, $P < .001$). The mean INR was 2.5. The percentage of maintenance time was 23% at a target INR of 2.0 or lower, 63% at a target INR of 2.1 to 3.0, 13% at a target INR of 3.1 to 4.0, and 1% at a target INR higher than 4.0.

The primary end point was any ischemic stroke, brain hemorrhage, or death from nonstroke vascular cause. The primary end point was reached in

22.1% of the aspirin group and 21.8% of the warfarin group. The probability of ischemic stroke in the territory of the stenotic artery at 1 year was 12% in the aspirin group and 11% in the warfarin group. At 2 years, the probabilities of ipsilateral ischemic stroke were 15% and 13%, respectively. Warfarin was associated with a higher rate of nonvascular death (1.1% versus 3.8%, $P = .05$) and major hemorrhage (3.2% versus 8.3%, $P = .02$). Data were nearly identical when analyzed by on-treatment analysis. The study was halted at the recommendation of the Data Safety and Monitoring Board because of excess mortality in the warfarin arm. The conclusion of the WASID trial was that aspirin should be preferred over warfarin for the treatment of symptomatic intracranial disease because of the lack of evidence for benefit with warfarin and lower risks of death and major bleeding with aspirin.

Subgroup analyses in the Warfarin versus Aspirin for Symptomatic Intracranial Disease trial

Prior retrospective studies had reported that certain subgroups of patients who have intracranial arterial stenosis are at particularly high risk of stroke. These subgroups include patients who had severe stenosis [20] or vertebrobasilar disease [21] or who did not respond to antithrombotic therapy [22]. The WASID trial provided a unique opportunity to determine prospectively whether these and other risk factors are associated with an increased risk of stroke in the territory of a stenotic intracranial artery. In a pooled analysis of all 569 patients in the WASID trial, ischemic stroke in any vascular territory occurred in 106 patients (19.0%); 77 (73%) of the strokes were in the territory of the stenotic artery [7]. In univariate analyses, severity of stenosis ($\geq 70\%$ versus $<70\%$), time from qualifying event to enrollment (≤ 17 days versus >17 days), female gender, score on the National Institutes of Health (NIH) stroke scale (>1 versus ≤ 1), and a history of diabetes mellitus were significantly associated ($P \leq .05$) with stroke in the territory of the stenotic artery; body mass index was of borderline significance ($P = .068$). Age, race, location of stenosis (ie, vertebrobasilar disease versus carotid-MCA disease), length of stenosis, other vascular risk factors, comorbidities, and treatment with antithrombotic agents at the time of the qualifying event (so-called "medical failures") were not significantly associated with an increased risk of stroke in the territory of the stenotic artery. Multivariate analysis showed that the only significant predictors of stroke in the territory were severity of stenosis ($\geq 70\%$ versus $<70\%$), time from qualifying event to enrollment (≤ 17 days versus >17 days), score on the NIH stroke scale (>1 versus ≤ 1), and female gender.

Severity of stenosis was the most powerful predictor of stroke in the territory and increased linearly (p-value for trend $=.0026$) with greater percent stenosis. The rates of stroke in the territory of the stenotic artery in patients who had a TIA or stroke and 70% or greater stenosis were 18% at 1 year (95% confidence interval [CI], 13%–24%) and 19% at 2 years (95% CI, 14%–25%), whereas the rates of stroke in the territory of the stenotic artery in patients who had a TIA or stroke and less than 70% stenosis were 6% at 1 year (95% CI, 4%–10%) and 10% at 2 years (95% CI, 7%–14%). Notably, two of the variables that previously had been associated with increased risk of stroke in retrospective studies, vertebrobasilar disease and lack of response to antithrombotic therapy, had no association with an increased risk for ipsilateral stroke. The current indication for the Wingspan device, which is approved by the FDA under a Humanitarian Device Exemption (HDE) for the treatment of intracranial stenosis, is for patients who have 50% to 99% stenosis and who have cerebral ischemic events during antithrombotic therapy. The data from the WASID trial do not support this requirement of failed antithrombotic therapy before using the Wingspan device.

Another important finding in the WASID trial was that 60 of the 77 strokes in the territory of the stenotic artery (78%) occurred within 1 year of enrollment. The magnitude of stroke risk and the temporal pattern of risk are nearly identical to data reported for the medical treatment arms of clinical trials for symptomatic extracranial carotid stenosis and occlusion [17,18]. Whether the decrease in stroke risk after 1 year reflects improvement in hemodynamic factors, embolic factors, or both over time is unclear.

A second subgroup analysis compared the outcomes with warfarin and aspirin in different subgroups of patients [8]. These subgroups were classified by time from qualifying event, age, gender, race, smoking, hypertension, diabetes, coronary artery disease, site of symptomatic lesion (middle cerebral, anterior cerebral, internal carotid, vertebral, and basilar arteries), anterior versus posterior circulation, per cent stenosis, length of stenosis, and antithrombotic therapy at the time of qualifying event. No definite differences in the risk of stroke or vascular death with aspirin or warfarin were observed in any of these subgroups, but the power of the study to detect differences in these subgroups was low.

In summary, angioplasty and stenting cannot be justified in patients who have stenosis of less than 70%, given the low risk of stroke in the territory of a stenotic artery (6% at 1 year) and the inherent risk of angioplasty and stenting (30-day rate of stroke and death in the range of 4%–7%, as discussed in the next section). Furthermore, lack of response to medical treatment should not be used as an indication for angioplasty and stenting. Patients in whom this procedure should be considered are those who have severe stenosis, recent ischemic symptoms, and a score on the NIH stroke scale greater than 1.

Medical management

Risk factor management in the WASID trial was performed by the study neurologist and primary care physicians, according to published national guidelines on hypertension [23], hyperlipidemia [24], and diabetes (American Diabetes Association) [25]. Despite these recommendations, many vascular risk factors were poorly controlled. Poorly controlled blood pressure and elevated low-density lipoprotein (LDL) levels were the most important risk factors for stroke, vascular death, or myocardial infarction during follow-up in WASID. During a mean of 1.8 years of follow-up, 30.7% of patients who had a mean systolic blood pressure of 140 mm Hg or higher had a stroke, vascular death, or myocardial infarction, compared with 18.3% of patients who had a mean systolic blood pressure lower than 140 mm Hg ($P < .0005$). Over the same period, 25.0% of patients who had LDL levels of 115 mg/dL (the median LDL) or higher had a stroke, vascular death, or myocardial infarction, compared with 18.6% of patients who had a mean LDL level below 115 mg/dL ($P = .03$). Considering an LDL target level of less than 70 mg/dL, 22.5% of patients who had a mean LDL above this target had a stroke, myocardial infarction, or vascular death, compared with 7.4% of those who had a mean LDL below this target (odds ratio 3.13; 95% CI, 0.77–12.67). Poorly controlled blood pressure and an elevated LDL level also were important risk factors for ischemic stroke alone in the WASID trial. The risk of any ischemic stroke was found to increase with increasing mean systolic blood pressure and diastolic blood pressure ($P < .0001$ and < 0.0001, respectively) using a log-rank trend test. Elevated systolic blood pressure and diastolic blood pressure also were associated with increased risk of ischemic stroke in the territory of the stenotic artery ($P = .0065$ and < 0.0001, respectively) [26]. An LDL of 115 mg/dL (the median value) or higher was highly correlated with ischemic stroke (odds ratio 1.82; 95% CI, 1.17–2.83; $P = .0072$) [27].

These risk factor data suggest that optimal outcome for patients who have intracranial atherosclerotic disease, including those who undergo angioplasty and stenting, requires careful and intensive adjunctive risk factor management. Further support for the importance of risk factor management in patients who have intracranial stenosis is provided by recent secondary prevention stroke trials that have shown treatment of elevated LDL [28] and blood pressure [29] reduces the risk of recurrent stroke. Additionally, intensive risk factor management in patients who have coronary artery disease has been shown to reduce major cardiac events and stroke [30,31] and to be as effective as endovascular intervention and usual or aggressive medical management for preventing cardiac ischemic events in patients who have stable angina and severe atherosclerotic coronary artery disease [32,33].

There are few data regarding the optimal antiplatelet regimen in this population. The WASID trial tested high-dose aspirin (1300 mg/d) and found it to be equivalent to warfarin in reducing the risk of stroke. There are no data on the effectiveness or safety of other antiplatelet agents specifically in patients who have intracranial stenosis. In other stroke populations with heterogeneous causes of stroke, the combination of aspirin and clopidogrel therapy was found to be equivalent to monotherapy in reducing the risk of stroke [34], and the combination of low-dose aspirin and dipyridamole has been shown to be more effective than low-dose aspirin for stroke prevention [35,36].

Angioplasty/stenting as a treatment for symptomatic intracranial stenosis

During the past decade, angioplasty and stenting have emerged as therapeutic options for symptomatic intracranial arterial stenosis. The first report of angioplasty for intracranial atherosclerotic disease was in 1980 [37]. Since then there have been dramatic improvements in balloon and stent technology and in the imaging systems that provide the guidance for these procedures.

Angioplasty alone

There have been no prospective studies of intracranial angioplasty without stent placement. Technical success (defined as reduction of stenosis to < 50%) can be achieved in more than 80% of patients, and the rate of stroke or death within 30 days of angioplasty has varied between 4% and 40% in several retrospective angioplasty studies [38–48]. One reason for the wide variation in complication rates may be variability in the acuity of patients being treated. Procedures that were largely elective were associated with lower complication rates (4%–6%) [43,44,46]. Restenosis rates following angioplasty alone range from 24% to 40% [43,44]. There are limited data on the long-term outcome after intracranial angioplasty alone. Marks and colleagues [43] reported an annual stroke rate of 4.4% (3.2%

in the territory of stenosis) in a recent retrospective review of 120 patients who underwent intracranial angioplasty at four sites. The actual stroke rate is uncertain, given the retrospective nature of the study and the lack of adjudication of events by neurologists. Although some practitioners strongly advocate the use of this procedure alone (ie, without a stent), most favor the use of stents. This preference can be attributed to several technical drawbacks to angioplasty, including immediate elastic recoil of the artery, dissection, acute vessel closure, residual stenosis of greater than 50% following the procedure, and high restenosis rates. These limitations, coupled with the success of stenting in the coronary circulation, have led to stenting becoming the preferred interventional technique for treating intracranial stenosis.

Stenting

Until recently, most data on the safety and efficacy of intracranial stenting have been limited to single-center series [49–59]. The largest of these studies are summarized in Table 1. These data suggest that intracranial stenting can be performed relatively safely and with high technical success. The larger, more recent studies suggest that the rate of stroke after stenting in patients who have 70% to 99% stenosis may be substantially lower than the rate of stroke in the patients who had equivalent stenosis in the WASID trial. Data exist for three categories of stents: bare-metal balloon expandable, drug-eluting balloon expandable, and self-expanding stents.

Balloon-expandable bare-metal stents

An industry-sponsored multicenter phase I trial of a balloon-expandable bare-metal stent (Neurolink, Guidant Corporation, St. Paul, MN) for intracranial stenosis provided encouraging data on the safety and potential efficacy of stenting for intracranial arterial stenosis. The Stenting of Symptomatic atherosclerotic Lesions in the Vertebral or Intracranial

Table 1: **Intracranial stenting case series**

Author	N	Vessel	Technical success	Major periprocedural complications	Follow-up period and events
Jiang et al [57]	42	ICA, MCA, VA, B	40/42 (95%)	4/42 (10%) "complication and death"	Median 8 months; 39 free of ischemic symptoms; restenosis 0/7 at 6 months, 0/4 at 12 months
Zhang et al [56]	48	ICA, MCA VA, B	46/48 (96%)	4/48 (8%): two vessel ruptures, one acute stent thrombosis, one perforate vessel occlusion	"short-term follow-up showed good clinical improvement"
Liu et al [55]	46	ICA, MCA VA, B	49/50 (98%)	1/46 (2%): one SAH (2%) extracranial carotid dissection requiring a stent	37/37 patients followed for a mean of 8.5 months were free of TIAs
de Rochemont et al [54]	18	ICA, MCA VA, B	18/20 (90%) stenoses	30-day combined stroke and death = 6%	0 recurrent events in 6 months
Jiang et al [58]	40	MCA	41/42 (98%)	3/40 (8%): three SAHs (one fatal); one acute occlusion treated with lytics without sequelae	Median 10 months; 0/38 had TIA or stroke; restenosis in 1/8 vessels
Lylyk et al [59]	106	ICA, MCA VA, B	104/106 (98%)	30-day stroke: 6/104 (5.7%); death: 4/104 (3.7%)	Restenosis in 7/58 (12%)

Abbreviations: B, basilar artery; ICA, internal carotid artery; MCA, middle cerebral artery; SAH, subarachnoid hemorrhage; TIA, transient ischemic attack; VA, vertebral artery.

Arteries (SSYLVIA) trial was a nonrandomized, multicenter study that evaluated the safety and performance of primary stenting in 43 patients who had intracranial arterial stenosis, 12 patients who had vertebral pre-PICA stenosis, and 6 patients who had vertebral ostium stenosis of 50% or greater [60]. Deployment of the stent was successful in 58 of the 61 patients (95%). In the first 30 days after stenting, 4 of 55 patients who had intracranial or pre-PICA stenosis (defined as "intracranial" in the WASID trial) had a stroke (30-day rate: 7.2%; 95% CI, 2.0%–17.6%); there were no deaths. The frequency of stroke within 1 year (including the 30-day rate) was 6 out of 55 (10.9%; 95% CI, 4.1%–22.3%). All strokes were in the territory of the treated artery. Recurrent stenosis of 50% or more at 6 months (intracranial, pre-PICA, and vertebral ostial lesions combined; data were not provided to separate out the vertebral ostial lesions) was documented by angiography in 18 of 51 patients (35%; 95% CI, 22.2%–48.4%).

Factors that were significantly associated with restenosis were diabetes, postprocedural diameter stenosis greater than 30%, and small vesseldiameter. These features also have been associated with higher rates of restenosis after coronary stenting. Of the 55 patients who had intracranial stenosis in the SSYLVIA trial, 33 had 70% to 99% stenosis. Of these 33 patients, 1 patient had a stroke within 30 days, and 2 patients had an ischemic stroke between day 31 and 1 year (Marcia Wachna, Guidant Corporation, personal communication, 2006). The SSYLVIA trial provides important preliminary pilot data suggesting that (1) intracranial stenting can be performed relatively safely (the point estimate of the 30-day stroke and death rate was similar to the 30-day stroke and death rate after carotid endarterectomy in the North American Symptomatic Carotid Endarterectomy Trial) [17]; (2) the risk of stroke at 1 year after stenting in patients who have 70% to 99% stenosis may be lower than the rate of stroke in similar patients in the WASID trial, suggesting a possible benefit of stenting in these high-risk patients. Based on these findings, Guidant Corporation applied to the FDA for approval of the Neurolink device for use in patients who do not respond to medical therapy, and an HDE was approved. Guidant Corporation has disbanded its Neurovascular Unit, however, and is no longer manufacturing the stent.

Another recent study by Jiang and colleagues [61] also suggests that the rate of stroke or symptomatic brain hemorrhage at 1 year after stenting in patients who have intracranial stenosis of 70% or more may be as low as 7.2%. This rate is substantially lower than the 1-year rate of stroke in patients who had stenosis of 70% or more in the WASID trial. The stent used in this study was a balloon-expandable stent that is not available in the United States.

Drug-eluting balloon expandable stents

Following the lead from cardiology, some investigators have treated patients who have intracranial stenosis with coronary drug-eluting stents that are not approved for the cerebral circulation and have not been shown to be safe in this population. The number of patients treated with drug-eluting stents for intracranial stenosis is too small to provide reliable data on the performance, safety, and potential efficacy of these stents in the cerebral circulation [62,63]. Preliminary experience indicates that these inflexible stents are difficult to deliver in the tortuous cerebral circulation, particularly to the MCAs, a common location of intracranial atherosclerosis. Additionally, it is likely that the future development of intracranial drug-eluting stents will be impeded by recent reports that coronary drug-eluting stents increase the risk of late-stent thrombosis and subsequent myocardial infarction or death [64] and that prolonged use of aspirin and clopidogrel is required with drug-eluting stents. The use of these drugs could increase the risk of major hemorrhage, particularly intracerebral hemorrhage [34].

Self-expanding stents

The bare metal self-expanding Wingspan stent (Boston Scientific) designed specifically to treat intracranial stenosis was approved by the FDA on August 3, 2005 for use under an HDE for patients who have intracranial stenosis "who are refractory to medical therapy." This approval was based on a European/Asian study of 45 patients who had symptomatic 50% to 99% stenosis and who had recurrent stroke on antithrombotic therapy. The main results of the study were that the stent was successfully deployed in 44 of 45 patients (98%) (95% CI, 88.2%–99.9%), the 30-day rate of stroke or death was 4.4% (95% CI, 0.5%–15.2%), and the 12-month rate of ipsilateral stroke or death was 9.3% (4/43) (95% CI, 2.6–22.1). Only 3 of 40 patients (7.5%) (95% CI, 1.6%–20.4%) had restenosis at 6 months, and none were symptomatic (www.fda.gov/cdrh/pdf5/h050001b.pdf). Of the 45 patients enrolled in the European/Asian Wingspan study, 29 had 70% to 99% stenosis. Of these 29 patients, 3 (10.3%) had a stroke in the territory or died with 1 year (95% CI, 2.2%–27.4%) [65].

More recently, Fiorella and colleagues [66] described their experience with the Wingspan device at four sites in the United States [67]. Seventy-eight patients who had symptomatic intracranial atherosclerotic stenosis were treated over a 9-month period. A total of 82 lesions were treated, 54 of which had stenosis of 70% or greater. Lesions treated involved the internal carotid (n = 32; 8 petrous; 10 cavernous; 11 supraclinoid segment; 3 terminus), vertebral (n = 14; V4 segment), basilar (n = 14), and middle cerebral (n = 22) arteries. The technical success rate was 98.8%; the mean pretreatment stenosis was 74.6%, and the mean poststent stenosis was 27.2%. There were five major periprocedural neurologic complications (two vessel perforations, both fatal; two ischemic strokes, both fatal; one nonfatal reperfusion hemorrhage) for an overall major periprocedural complication rate of 6.1%.

Priority for a trial

The stage is optimally set for a randomized trial comparing stenting with medical therapy because a series of events have converged:

1. Completion of the WASID trial has enabled identification of patients at high risk of stroke despite usual medical management.
2. Completion of two phase I trials have established preliminary safety and feasibility of intracranial stenting for patients who have intracranial stenosis.
3. The FDA has approved the Wingspan intracranial stent under an HDE for treating patients who have failed antithrombotic therapy.
4. Boston Scientific has conducted training in the use of the Wingspan stent and delivery system in more 50 sites in the United States.
5. There has been accumulating experience with Wingspan in clinical practice.
6. The results of antihypertensive and recent lipid-lowering therapy trials mandate an evaluation of the role of aggressive risk factor management in patients who have intracranial stenosis, a particularly high-risk subtype of cerebrovascular disease.

Because the Wingspan is the only FDA-approved stent for intracranial atherosclerotic stenosis and is likely to remain so for the next several years, given the length of time required to develop and test new stents and to receive FDA approval, it now is incumbent on investigators to determine the efficacy of stenting with Wingspan before it becomes established as standard but unproven as therapy for intracranial stenosis.

Summary

Symptomatic atherosclerotic intracranial stenosis is a high-risk condition. The recently completed WASID trial has provided excellent estimates of the outcome of these patients treated with aspirin or warfarin and usual management of risk factors. Angioplasty and stenting cannot be justified in patients who have less than 70% stenosis, given the low risk of stroke in the territory of a stenotic artery (6% at 1 year) and the inherent risk of current technology. Furthermore, failure to respond to medical treatment should not be required as an indication for angioplasty and stenting. Women who have severe stenosis, recent ischemic symptoms, an NIH stroke scale score greater than 1 are at the highest risk for stroke and therefore have the greatest likelihood of benefiting from angioplasty and stenting. The linear relationship between the degree of stenosis and stroke risk with medical therapy also supports a mechanical approach to revascularization. At present, however, there is no level 1 evidence to support angioplasty and stenting for patients who have symptomatic intracranial atherosclerotic disease. Case series suggest that the safety and stroke risk reduction of this procedure may provide a benefit, particularly with self-expanding stent technology. A randomized, controlled trial is needed to prove the efficacy of this therapy. It also should be noted that these patients as a group frequently have vascular risk factors and require aggressive medical management. In addition, rates of restenosis and the clinical consequences of restenosis must be monitored closely in future studies. Advances in stent design may be required if self-expanding bare-metal stents are associated with a high risk of stroke resulting from restenosis in clinical trials.

References

[1] Sacco RL, Kargman DE, Gu Q, et al. Race-ethnicity and determinants of intracranial atherosclerotic cerebral infarction. Stroke 1995;26:14–20.
[2] Wityk RJ, Lehman D, Klag M, et al. Race and sex differences in the distribution of cerebral atherosclerosis. Stroke 1996;27:1974–80.
[3] Feldmann E, Daneault N, Kwan E, et al. Chinese-white differences in the distribution of occlusive cerebrovascular disease. Neurology 1990;40:1541–5.
[4] Chimowitz MI, Lynn MJ, Howlett-Smith H, et al. Comparison of warfarin and aspirin for symptomatic intracranial arterial stenosis. N Engl J Med 2005;352:1305–16.
[5] Grubb RL Jr, Derdeyn CP, Fritsch SM, et al. Importance of hemodynamic factors in the prognosis of symptomatic carotid occlusion. JAMA 1998;280:1055–60.
[6] Caplan LR, Hennerici M. Impaired clearance of emboli (washout) is an important link between hypoperfusion, embolism, and ischemic stroke. Arch Neurol 1998;55:1475–82.
[7] Kasner SE, Chimowitz MI, Lynn MJ, et al. Predictors of ischemic stroke in the territory of a symptomatic intracranial arterial stenosis. Circulation 2006;113:555–63.

[8] Kasner SE, Lynn MJ, Chimowitz MI, et al. Warfarin vs aspirin for symptomatic intracranial stenosis: subgroup analyses from WASID. Neurology 2006;67:1275–8.

[9] Benesch CG, Chimowitz MI. Best treatment for intracranial arterial stenosis? 50 years of uncertainty. The WASID investigators. Neurology 2000;55:465–6.

[10] Broderick J, Brott T, Kothari R, et al. The Greater Cincinnati/Northern Kentucky Stroke Study: preliminary first-ever and total incidence rates of stroke among blacks. Stroke 1998;29:415–21.

[11] Executive Committee of the Asymptomatic Carotid Atherosclerosis Study. Endarterectomy for asymptomatic carotid artery stenosis. JAMA 1995;273:1421–8.

[12] Hart RG, Halperin JL. Atrial fibrillation and thromboembolism: a decade of progress in stroke prevention. Ann Intern Med 1999;131:688–95.

[13] Derdeyn CP, Powers WJ, Grubb RL Jr. Hemodynamic effects of middle cerebral artery stenosis and occlusion. AJNR Am J Neuroradiol 1998;19:1463–9.

[14] Yamauchi H, Fukuyama H, Nagahama Y, et al. Significance of increased oxygen extraction fraction in five-year prognosis of major cerebral arterial occlusive disease. J Nucl Med 1999;40:1992–8.

[15] Lee DK, Kim JS, Kwon SU, et al. Lesion patterns and stroke mechanism in atherosclerotic middle cerebral artery disease: early diffusion-weighted imaging study. Stroke 2005;36:2583–8.

[16] Amin-Hanjani S, Du X, Zhao M, et al. Use of quantitative magnetic resonance angiography to stratify stroke risk in symptomatic vertebrobasilar disease. Stroke 2005;36:1140–5.

[17] North American Symptomatic Carotid Endarterectomy Trial (NASCET) Collaborators. Beneficial effect of carotid endarterectomy in symptomatic patients with high-grade carotid stenosis. N Engl J Med 1991;325:445–53.

[18] The EC/IC Bypass Study Group. Failure of extracranial-intracranial arterial bypass to reduce the risk of ischemic stroke: Results of an international randomized trial. N Engl J Med 1985;313:1191–2000.

[19] Samuels OB, Joseph GJ, Lynn MJ, et al. A standardized method for measuring intracranial arterial stenosis. AJNR Am J Neuroradiol 2000;21:643–6.

[20] Chimowitz MI, Kokkinos J, Strong J, et al. The warfarin-aspirin symptomatic intracranial disease study. Neurology 1995;45:1488–93.

[21] The Warfarin-Aspirin Symptomatic Intracranial Disease (WASID) study group. Prognosis of patients with symptomatic vertebral or basilar artery stenosis. Stroke 1998;29:1389–92.

[22] Thijs VN, Albers GW. Symptomatic intracranial atherosclerosis: outcome of patients who fail antithrombotic therapy. Neurology 2000;55:490–7.

[23] Chobanian AV, Bakris GL, Black HR, et al. The seventh report of the Joint National Committee On Prevention, Detection, Evaluation, And Treatment of High Blood Pressure: the JNC 7 report. JAMA 2003;289:2560–72.

[24] Grundy SM, Cleeman JI, Merz CN, et al. Implications of recent clinical trials for the National Cholesterol Education Program Adult Treatment Panel III guidelines. Circulation 2004;110:227–39.

[25] Standards of medical care in diabetes–2006. Diabetes Care 2006;29(Suppl 1):S4–42.

[26] Circulation in press.

[27] Turan TN, Cotsonis GA, Lynn MJ, et al. Risk factors associated with recurrent ischemic stroke in patients with symptomatic intracranial stenosis. Presented at the Joint World Congress of Stroke. Cape Town, South Africa, October 27, 2006.

[28] Amarenco P, Bogousslavsky J, Callahan A 3rd, et al. High-dose atorvastatin after stroke or transient ischemic attack. N Engl J Med 2006;355:549–59.

[29] Randomised trial of a perindopril-based blood-pressure-lowering regimen among 6,105 individuals with previous stroke or transient ischaemic attack. Lancet 2001;358:1033–41.

[30] Sacks FM, Pfeffer MA, Moye LA, et al. for the Cholesterol and Recurrent Events Trial Investigators. The effect of pravastatin on coronary events after myocardial infarction in patients with average cholesterol levels. N Engl J Med 1996;335:1001–9.

[31] Scandinavian Simvastatin Survival Study Group. Randomized trial of cholesterol lowering in 4444 patients with coronary artery disease. The Scandinavian Simvastatin Survival Study (4S). Lancet 1994;344:1383–9.

[32] Pitt B, Waters D, Brown WV, et al. Atorvastatin versus revascularization treatment investigators. Aggressive lipid-lowering therapy compared with angioplasty in stable coronary artery disease. N Engl J Med 1999;341:70–6.

[33] Boden WE, O'Rourke RA, Teo KK, et al. the CTRG. Optimal medical therapy with or without pci for stable coronary disease. N Engl J Med 2007;356(15):1503–16.

[34] Diener PH-C, Bogousslavsky PJ, Brass PLM, et al. Aspirin and clopidogrel compared with clopidogrel alone after recent ischaemic stroke or transient ischaemic attack in high-risk patients (match): randomised, double-blind, placebo-controlled trial. Lancet 2004;364:331–7.

[35] Diener HC, Cunha L, Forbes C, et al. European Stroke Prevention Study. 2. Dipyridamole and acetylsalicylic acid in the secondary prevention of stroke. J Neurol Sci 1996;143:1–13.

[36] ESPRIT Study Group: Halkes PH, van Gijn J, Kappelle LJ, et al. Aspirin plus dipyridamole versus aspirin alone after cerebral ischaemia of arterial origin (esprit): randomised controlled trial. Lancet 367:1665–73.

[37] Sundt TM Jr, Smith HC, Campbell JK, et al. Transluminal angioplasty for basilar artery stenosis. Mayo Clin Proc 1980;55:673–80.

[38] Higashida RT, Tsai FY, Halbach VV, et al. Transluminal angioplasty for atherosclerotic disease of the vertebral and basilar arteries. J Neurosurg 1993;78:192–8.

[39] Clark WM, Barnwell SL, Nesbit G, et al. Safety and efficacy of percutaneous transluminal angioplasty for intracranial atherosclerotic stenosis. Stroke 1995;26:1200–4.

[40] Tuoho H. Percutaneous transluminal angioplasty in the treatment of atherosclerotic disease in the anterior circulation and hemodynamic evaluation. J Neurosurg 1995;82:953–60.

[41] Takis C, Kwan ES, Pessin MS, et al. Intracranial angioplasty: experience and complications. AJNR Am J Neuroradiol 1997;18:1661–8.

[42] Marks MP, Marcellus M, Norbash AM, et al. Outcome of angioplasty for atherosclerotic intracranial stenosis. Stroke 1999;30:1065–9.

[43] Marks MP, Wojak JC, Al-Ali F, et al. Angioplasty for symptomatic intracranial stenosis: clinical outcome. Stroke 2006;37:1016–20.

[44] Connors JJ 3rd, Wojak JC. Percutaneous transluminal angioplasty for intracranial atherosclerotic lesions: evolution of technique and short-term results. J Neurosurg 1999;91:415–23.

[45] Alazzaz A, Thornton J, Aletich VA, et al. Intracranial percutaneous transluminal angioplasty for arteriosclerotic stenosis. Arch Neurol 2000;57:1625–30.

[46] Nahser HC, Henkes H, Weber W, et al. Intracranial vertebrobasilar stenosis: angioplasty and follow-up. AJNR Am J Neuroradiol 2000;21:1293–301.

[47] Gress DR, Smith WS, Dowd CF, et al. Angioplasty for intracranial symptomatic vertebrobasilar ischemia. Neurosurgery 2002;51:23–7 [discussion: 27–9].

[48] Gupta R, Schumacher HC, Mangla S, et al. Urgent endovascular revascularization for symptomatic intracranial atherosclerotic stenosis. Neurology 2003;61:1729–35.

[49] Gomez CR, Misra VK, Campbell MS, et al. Elective stenting of symptomatic middle cerebral artery stenosis. AJNR Am J Neuroradiol 2000;21:971–3.

[50] Gomez CR, Misra VK, Liu MW, et al. Elective stenting of symptomatic basilar artery stenosis. Stroke 2000;31:95–9.

[51] Rasmussen PA, Perl J 2nd, Barr JD, et al. Stent-assisted angioplasty of intracranial vertebrobasilar atherosclerosis: an initial experience. J Neurosurg 2000;92:771–8.

[52] Levy EI, Hanel RA, Boulos AS, et al. Comparison of periprocedure complications resulting from direct stent placement compared with those due to conventional and staged stent placement in the basilar artery. J Neurosurg 2003;99:653–60.

[53] Kim DJ, Lee BH, Kim DI, et al. Stent-assisted angioplasty of symptomatic intracranial vertebrobasilar artery stenosis: feasibility and follow-up results. AJNR Am J Neuroradiol 2005;26:1381–8.

[54] de Rochemont M, Turowski B, Buchkremer M, et al. Recurrent symptomatic high-grade intracranial stenoses: safety and efficacy of undersized stents—initial experience. Radiology 2004;231:45–9.

[55] Liu JM, Hong B, Huang QH, et al. [Safety and short-term results of stent-assisted angioplasty for the treatment of intracranial arterial stenosis]. Zhonghua Wai Ke Za Zhi 2004;42:169–72 [in Chinese].

[56] Zhang QZ, Miao ZR, Li SM, et al. [Complications of stent-assistant angioplasty of symptomatic intracranial artery stenosis]. Zhonghua Yi Xue Za Zhi 2003;83:1402–5 [in Chinese].

[57] Jiang WJ, Du B, Wang YJ, et al. [Symptomatic intracranial artery stenosis: angiographic classifications and stent-assisted angioplasty]. Zhonghua Nei Ke Za Zhi 2003;42:545–9 [in Chinese].

[58] Jiang WJ, Wang YJ, Du B, et al. Stenting of symptomatic m1 stenosis of middle cerebral artery: an initial experience of 40 patients. Stroke 2004;35:1375–80.

[59] Lylyk P, Vila JF, Miranda C, et al. Endovascular reconstruction by means of stent placement in symptomatic intracranial atherosclerotic stenosis. Neurol Res 2005;27(Suppl 1):S84–8.

[60] SSYLVIA Study Investigators. Stenting of Symptomatic Atherosclerotic Lesions in the Vertebral or Intracranial Arteries (SSYLVIA): study results. Stroke 2004;35:1388–92.

[61] Jiang WJ, Xu XT, Du B, et al. Comparison of elective stenting of severe vs moderate intracranial atherosclerotic stenosis. Neurology 2007;68:420–6.

[62] Gupta R, Al-Ali F, Thomas AJ, et al. Safety, feasibility, and short-term follow-up of drug-eluting stent placement in the intracranial and extracranial circulation. Stroke 2006;37:2562–6.

[63] Abou-Chebl A, Bashir Q, Yadav JS. Drug-eluting stents for the treatment of intracranial atherosclerosis: initial experience and midterm angiographic follow-up. Stroke 2005;36:e165–8.

[64] Iakovou I, Schmidt T, Bonizzoni E, et al. Incidence, predictors, and outcome of thrombosis after successful implantation of drug-eluting stents. JAMA 2005;293:2126–30.

[65] Hartmann M, Bose A, Henkes H, et al. One year stroke risks in high grade, symptomatic, medically refractory intracranial atherosclerosis after angioplasty and stenting: the Wingspan trial. Presented at the International Stroke Conference. Kissimmee (FL), February 18, 2006.

[66] Fiorella D, Levy EI, Turk AS, et al. US multicenter experience with the Wingspan stent system for the treatment of intracranial atheromatous disease: periprocedural results. Stroke 2007;38:881–7.

[67] Henkes H, Miloslavski E, Lowens S, et al. Treatment of intracranial atherosclerotic stenoses with balloon dilatation and self-expanding stent deployment (Wingspan). Neuroradiology 2005;47:222–8.

ELSEVIER
SAUNDERS

NEUROIMAGING
CLINICS
OF NORTH AMERICA

Neuroimag Clin N Am 17 (2007) 365–380

Technique for Intracranial Balloon and Stent-Assisted Angioplasty for Atherosclerotic Stenosis

DeWitte T. Cross, III, MD[a,b,*], Christopher J. Moran, MD[a,b],
Colin P. Derdeyn, MD[a,b,c]

- Patient selection
- Timing of the procedure
- Patient preparation
- Anesthesia
- Access
- Guiding catheters and sheaths
- Baseline angiography
- Anticoagulation
- Balloon versus stent-assisted angioplasty decision
- Dilation device selection
- Wire selection
- Advancement and positioning of dilation device
- Dilation
- Assessment
- Further dilation
- Complications
- Postprocedure management
- Follow-up
- Re-treatment
- Summary
- Further readings

Patient selection

Elsewhere in this issue, the benefits and risks associated with endovascular treatment of intracranial atherosclerotic stenosis are weighed. In general, a patient selected for this procedure is one who has symptoms of transient ischemic attack (TIA) or stroke related to the target lesion, who has failed a trial of antiplatelet or anticoagulant therapy, and who has a stenosis that can be reached and dilated with reasonable safety using currently available devices. Stenoses of the larger arteries, such as the distal internal carotid artery, distal vertebral artery, basilar artery, and proximal middle cerebral artery, typically are dilated, rather than those of the smaller or more distal vessels. Although MR angiography or CT angiography screening examinations may identify an intracranial stenosis, conventional angiographic assessment of the stenosis should be performed at some point before treatment, not only to define the target lesion better, but to assess further the route to be taken to reach the stenosis with catheters and devices. The findings of the conventional angiogram, MR or CT imaging studies, and the history and clinical examination can be presented and discussed at a multidisciplinary conference to arrive at

[a] Washington University School of Medicine, 510 South Kingshighway Boulevard, Box 8131, St. Louis, MO 63110, USA
[b] Barnes-Jewish Hospital and St. Louis Children's Hospital, Washington University School of Medicine, 510 South Kingshighway Boulevard, Box 8131, St. Louis, MO 63110, USA
[c] Washington University School of Medicine, Mallinckrodt Institute of Radiology, Department of Neurology and Neurological Surgery, 510 South Kingshighway Blvd., St. Louis, MO 63110, USA
* Corresponding author. Radiology and Neurological Surgery, Washington University School of Medicine, 510 South Kingshighway Boulevard, Box 8131, St. Louis, MO 63110.
E-mail address: crossde@wustl.edu (D.T. Cross).

Timing of the procedure

For a patient having infrequent, related TIAs, a procedure to dilate a symptomatic intracranial arterial stenosis can be performed electively, when antiplatelet pretreatment is optimized and warfarin, if prescribed, has been discontinued far enough in advance so as to be ineffective at the time of the procedure. For a patient having frequent or "crescendo" TIAs, the procedure can be performed urgently. In such a situation, antiplatelet drugs can be given with loading doses (see later discussion) if a patient has not been maintained on those drugs in the week before the procedure. Warfarin can be reversed by intravenous administration of fresh frozen plasma, for an urgent procedure.

For a patient with a related acute stroke who is stable or improving following initial presentation, the procedure can be scheduled after a 4- to 6-week period of medical therapy to reduce the risk of hemorrhagic transformation of the infarction or hemorrhage related to a perfusion pressure breakthrough phenomenon. For a patient with an acute stroke who is continuing to decline as a result of extension of the infarction or rethrombosis at a site of stenosis, dilation of the stenosis is sometimes performed emergently as an adjunct to intra-arterial thrombolysis within the time frame observed for use of lytic drugs in acute stroke (usually within 6 hours of symptom onset in the carotid circulation, or longer in the case of basilar thrombosis).

Patient preparation

An elective patient is usually pretreated (assuming no aspirin allergy) with a combination of aspirin and a second antiplatelet drug to lower the risk of a thromboembolic complication during or after the procedure. Aspirin reaches full effectiveness in most patients within 1 to 2 hours of an oral dose, so timing of the initiation of aspirin pretreatment is not as critical as for the second drug. Aspirin is usually given as 325 mg orally per day. Clopidogrel is the most commonly used and preferred second antiplatelet drug, based on experience from coronary interventions. Clopidogrel, given as 75 mg orally per day, the routine maintenance dose, should be started 5 days in advance of the procedure to reach full effectiveness. A common pretreatment regimen for elective patients is thus, aspirin, 325 mg, and clopidogrel, 75 mg, orally per day beginning 5 days before treatment and including the morning of treatment.

For patients allergic to aspirin, aspirin is omitted. For patients allergic to clopidogrel, other options exist. Cilostazol, 100 mg orally twice daily (taken on an empty stomach), can be substituted for clopidogrel. A combination of aspirin, 25 mg, and dipyridamole, 200 mg, one capsule orally twice daily, can be also substituted for clopidogrel and the additional aspirin dose decreased from 325 to 81 mg daily. Headache and gastrointestinal side effects are more common with cilostazol and dipyridamole than with clopidogrel. Ticlopidine, 250 mg orally twice daily (taken with food), is another substitute for clopidogrel, but patients must be periodically checked for thrombocytopenia as a side effect of the drug.

For urgent procedures, a routine 325-mg dose of aspirin is given before the procedure, and clopidogrel is given with a loading dose of 300 to 450 mg, administered at least 6 hours before the procedure, if possible. For emergent procedures, intravenous antiplatelet agents can be given in place of the oral antiplatelet agents at considerably greater cost. Abciximab for central nervous system (CNS) use can be given as a 0.20 mg/kg IV bolus immediately before the intervention, with the maintenance IV drip of 0.125 mcg/kg/min (maximum 10 mcg/min) for 12 hours as an option during and after the procedure. Alternatively, eptifibatide can be given as two IV boluses of 180 mcg/kg (maximum 22.6 mg) administered 10 minutes apart, with the maintenance IV drip of 2 mcg/kg/min (maximum 15 mg/hr) for 12 hours as an option during and after treatment.

Warfarin is usually discontinued 3 to 4 days before an elective procedure to allow the international normalized ratio (INR) to fall into a normal range at the time of treatment. For patients judged to be dependent on systemic anticoagulation (eg, for those in atrial fibrillation with left atrial enlargement at risk for cardiogenic embolism), heparin anticoagulation can be initiated when the INR falls below a therapeutic range. For urgent or emergent procedures, fresh-frozen plasma can be given to reverse the effects of warfarin.

Anesthesia

Although angioplasty and stent deployment in the thoracic and cervical segments of the carotid and vertebral arteries are performed commonly with moderate procedural sedation, dilation of more fragile intracranial arteries is performed best under general anesthesia. Not only does general anesthesia allow optimal imaging and sizing of a stenosis, it allows stable road mapping, proper wire navigation, and accurate device positioning (Fig. 1). Pharmacologic paralysis prevents patient motion from occurring at critical times in the procedure, such

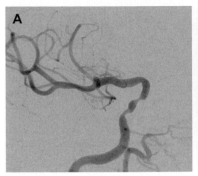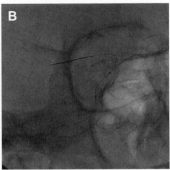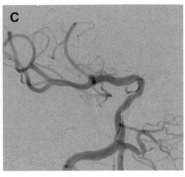

Fig. 1. Angioplasty and stenting for a symptomatic petrous segment right internal carotid artery stenosis. This patient was a 62-year-old man with a recent right parietal stroke. At the time of treatment, he had daily limb-shaking TIAs on warfarin. The right middle cerebral artery appeared isolated, without collateral sources of flow from the circle of Willis. (*A*) Working projection after a right common carotid artery injection. The procedure was performed under general anesthesia. A long 6F sheath was placed into the right internal carotid artery from a femoral approach. (*B*) A 3.5 mm × 12 mm stent placed primarily over a 0.014 in wire. (*C*) Angiography after stent placement, showing minimal residual stenosis and no distal emboli.

as during the slow, gentle dilation step, when a temporary reduction in cerebral perfusion might lead to confusion or agitation on the part of the patient. Perforation or rupture of an intracranial artery during dilation could result in a neurologically catastrophic or fatal complication, and the chance of this perforation or rupture occurring is minimized by removing patient motion from the equation with general anesthesia.

Another advantage of general anesthesia is better control of systemic blood pressure during, and immediately after, arterial dilation. Certain patients depend on pial collateral flow to maintain adequate cerebral perfusion in the territory distal to a stenosis, and, with impaired autoregulation, may depend on mildly elevated systemic mean arterial pressures to feed the pial collateral network adequately. Before the dilation of a stenosis in such a situation, it is desirable to maintain mean arterial pressures at the patient's baseline. After a successful dilation, in the setting of impaired autoregulation, it is desirable to lower the mean arterial pressure into a normotensive range to avoid potential perfusion pressure breakthrough effects, particularly if the patient has had a recent infarction in the territory of the stenosis. The anesthesiologist can begin intravenous infusions of drugs such as phenylephrine to raise pressure if necessary after induction, or nicarpidine to lower pressure after dilation, for prolonged effects, or adjust delivery rates of anesthetic agents, or administer other drugs for short-term effects on systemic pressures.

Access

The standard femoral arterial approach works well in most cases, but arterial anatomy defined by the aortic arch injection and catheterization experience from the diagnostic cerebral angiogram may indicate that an alternative access approach would work better. If it is difficult to place a diagnostic cerebral catheter in an artery from a femoral approach, it will be even more difficult to advance a relatively stiff stent delivery balloon catheter against the resistance of vessel tortuosity to achieve success in distal navigation and delivery through that artery. Choice of access site is a concern for target stenoses in the posterior circulation more often than for those in the anterior circulation in actual practice.

If the target stenosis is in a distal vertebral artery, close attention should be paid to the anatomy of the proximal vertebral artery to decide on the access approach. In the special situation in which the vertebral artery arises from the aorta directly and is of too small a diameter to accept a guide, a femoral approach would still be taken, but the guiding catheter or sheath chosen would need to be one that offered the best possible stability in the aortic arch. In the situation in which the origin of the vertebral artery from the subclavian artery is more parallel to the distal subclavian than to the proximal subclavian artery, a brachial approach would offer better stability and would be preferable to a femoral approach (**Fig. 2**). A brachial approach might also be better for situations in which the aorta is ectatic and tortuous or in which the proximal subclavian artery is diseased, even if the vertebral origin is perpendicular to the subclavian curve, because the length of the guiding catheter in the body is reduced when a brachial approach is used. If the target stenosis is in the basilar artery, the approach taken to reach the stenosis is usually through the dominant vertebral artery, unless that distal vertebral artery is

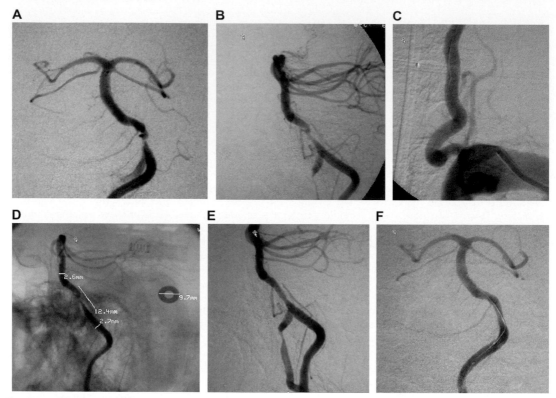

Fig. 2. Brachial approach for angioplasty and stenting for a symptomatic basilar artery stenosis. This patient was a 75-year-old man with recurrent posterior circulation TIAs on anti-platelet therapy, including diplopia. Posteroanterior (*A*) and lateral (*B*) working projections after a left vertebral artery injection. No collateral flow was present from either posterior communicating artery. Initially, a long 7F sheath was placed in the left subclavian artery near the vertebral artery origin from a femoral approach. A balloon-expandable coronary stent could not be advanced across the stenosis even though a 300 cm 0.014 in exchange wire had been placed across the stenosis via microcatheter. A 6F guide catheter was then introduced from a left brachial approach and positioned at the left vertebral artery origin. (*C*) Measurements of the stenotic segment prior to treatment. (*D*) A 2.5 mm × 8 mm stent was successfully deployed primarily across the stenosis from this approach over a standard 0.014 in wire. Post-angioplasty result in lateral (*E*) and posteroanterior (*F*) projections.

more diseased than the nondominant vertebral artery, and the access approach chosen, femoral or brachial, should be one that is optimal for catheterizing that proximal vertebral artery.

Sometimes, extreme tortuosity of the brachiocephalic arteries hinders catheterization of the cervical carotid artery. If the target stenosis is in the carotid territory and placement of a stable guiding catheter or sheath is impossible from a femoral approach, a brachial approach to carotid catheterization and an exchange for a guiding catheter can be attempted, as can a direct cervical common carotid artery puncture for placement of a short arterial sheath. Using a direct carotid approach leads to the issue of achieving hemostasis after removal of the sheath. Compressing a carotid artery in which a stent has just been placed distally risks diminishing distal flow and local hematoma development, particularly if the patient remains heparin-anticoagulated, so an alternative to compression is having a neurosurgeon or vascular surgeon remove the sheath and oversew the arterial defect after the procedure.

Guiding catheters and sheaths

One of the most important aspects of a successful procedure is establishing a stable catheterization of the parent artery. It is assumed that the reader has knowledge of, and experience with, catheterizing common carotid and vertebral arteries using standard cerebral catheters and guidewires.

For a target stenosis in a distal internal carotid or proximal middle cerebral artery to be treated from a femoral approach, the ideal platform is a firm guiding catheter or sheath with a soft and flexible tip that is positioned in the upper cervical internal carotid artery. Softer guide catheters (eg, 5 French

Envoy, Cordis, Miami, FL) typically used for other interventional neuroradiologic procedures for placement of very flexible and trackable microcatheters may not provide the degree of support necessary for delivery of less flexible balloon or stent delivery catheters. Such small-diameter, soft guide catheters may be pushed back into the aorta by forward force applied to relatively stiff device catheters within them. More suitable guides for intracranial angioplasty or stent delivery are slightly larger, with sturdier walls (eg, 6 French Guider, Target Therapeutics/Boston Scientific, Fremont, CA, for less tortuous routes, or the 80-cm long 6 French Shuttle sheath, Cook, Inc., Bloominton, IN). Even more support is sometimes necessary, and in those cases, a 6F guiding catheter can be placed coaxially within a 6F guiding sheath. One should always check the minimum inner diameter guiding catheter required for the intended stent delivery system and be certain the guiding catheter chosen has an inner diameter large enough to be compatible with it.

Placement of the guiding catheter or sheath in a carotid artery is usually performed by exchanging the diagnostic catheter over an exchange wire for the guide. In most situations, this exchange can be performed with the diagnostic catheter and exchange wire positioned in the upper cervical common carotid artery, to avoid inducing vasospasm in the internal carotid artery. Most often, a standard 3-mm J exchange wire will suffice, but in cases in which tortuosity might interfere with the catheter exchange in the common carotid artery and more wire support is needed, the diagnostic catheter can be advanced into the external carotid artery and the exchange wire can be advanced out an external carotid branch. In such cases, an exchange wire with a flexible hydrophilic tip and firmer principal wire (eg, Connors, Cook, Inc.) is useful. If an arterial sheath has been placed in the femoral artery during initial access, it will need to be of a sufficient size to allow passage of the chosen guide catheter (eg, 6F for a 6F guiding catheter), but will need to be removed over the exchange wire along with the diagnostic catheter if a guiding sheath (eg, 6 French Shuttle) is chosen for placement in the parent artery. Once the guiding catheter or sheath is delivered over the exchange wire into the distal common carotid artery, it can be advanced over a hydrophilic wire (eg, Roadrunner, Cook, Inc.) into the cervical internal carotid using a road map. Advancing the guide or sheath as far as possible into the cervical internal carotid artery will offer the best support, but care should be taken not to advance any portion of a relatively stiff sheath, its inner dilator, or a guiding catheter into the petrous internal carotid artery, to avoid dissecting the vessel.

If the proximal internal carotid artery is too sharply angled relative to the common carotid artery (eg, at a 90° angle to each other), or if there is atherosclerotic stenosis of any significant degree at the internal carotid artery origin, the guiding sheath or catheter is left in the distal common carotid artery.

For a target stenosis in the distal vertebral artery or basilar artery, the caliber of the vertebral artery, the origin of the vertebral artery, and the access site chosen will influence the choice of guiding catheter and placement steps. A small-to-medium–diameter vertebral artery may limit the guiding catheter to a 5F size (eg, Envoy), whereas a 6F guide catheter can be used in a large vertebral artery. A larger, stiffer guiding sheath (eg, 6 French Shuttle) generally is not used in a vertebral artery proper, but may be very appropriate if the guiding catheter tip must be positioned in the subclavian artery or aortic arch just proximal to the vertebral artery origin. Guiding catheters larger than 5F generally are not necessary or used from a brachial approach.

Placing a guide catheter in a vertebral artery from a femoral approach is often done as an exchange for a diagnostic catheter over an exchange wire, similar to the steps described earlier for placement of a carotid guide. The exchange wire in the smaller vertebral artery is generally a straight-tipped or 1-mm J-tipped wire, rather than the 3-mm J-tipped wire. From a brachial approach, or from a femoral approach with very little tortuosity, the guide catheter can be placed primarily over an angled wire. A good combination for primary guide catheter placement, for example, is a 90-cm–long 5F Envoy catheter in which a 100-cm–long 4F Cordis H1 catheter has been placed coaxially hub to hub, directed over a Cook 0.035-in Roadrunner wire, advanced using a road map for optimal positioning. The 4F inner catheter tip protrudes a few millimeters outside the guide catheter tip, is used to help direct the wire and guide catheter into the vertebral artery origin, and serves to smooth the transition from the diameter of the wire to the guide catheter in this more fragile artery. (Note that the 4.1F Cook diagnostic catheters will not fit coaxially within the 5F Envoy catheters.) As in the carotid artery, the further the guide catheter can be advanced into the cervical vertebral artery, the more stable the system will be, but kinks, turns, or stenoses in the proximal vertebral artery may limit advancement. The guide catheter should not be forced through acutely angled vessel segments, or further superiorly than the horizontal turn of the vertebral artery at C2, to avoid dissecting the vessel or inducing vasospasm that would obstruct flow. Once the guide catheter is positioned, any coaxial catheter is removed. (Because there is no flush around the 4F catheter within the 5F guide, the catheterization with that coaxial system should be performed gently but without delay, and the guide catheter should be aspirated and flushed, as would be the case after any guide catheter placement.)

A test injection of contrast into the guiding catheter or sheath following final positioning should be performed to be certain the maneuvers to place it did not induce significant vasospasm in the internal carotid artery or vertebral artery before proceeding. If significant vasospasm is seen, it may be necessary to withdraw the guide slightly, wait several minutes until the vasospasm resolves, or treat the vasospasm with intra-arterial drugs (eg, papaverine, 1–10 mL of a 3 mg/mL solution, or verapamil, 1–10 mL of a 1 mg/mL solution, in normal saline given at 1 mL/min or slower, so as not to lower systemic arterial pressure).

Baseline angiography

Initial angiography performed during the procedure, after placement of a diagnostic cerebral catheter, guiding catheter, or sheath in the parent artery, is performed to define the stenosis, to measure the diameter of the artery accurately at the stenosis and in nondiseased arterial segments immediately proximal and distal to the stenosis, and to measure the length of the stenosis to be treated. The arterial tree distal to the stenosis is imaged in standard projections to compare distal branches before and after treatment of the stenosis, to identify any emboli that might result, and the stenosis is examined in a sufficient number of projections to define optimal working projections for navigation of a balloon or stent delivery catheter and its wire. If the angiographic unit does not have a built-in calibration and vessel-measurement system, reference markers may be placed on the head for calibration of the angiographic measurements. Some wires have calibration markers that can also be used to measure the length of a stenosis if placed in the field of view. As a final check on the validity of the measurements, one should be aware that the diameter of the average internal carotid artery is approximately 5 mm in the petrous segment and approximately 4 mm in the supraclinoid segment, the diameter of the average proximal middle cerebral artery (the M1 segment) is approximately 2.7 to 3.0 mm, and the diameter of the average basilar artery is approximately 3 mm.

Anticoagulation

Systemic anticoagulation can be initiated following placement of the arterial sheath or guide catheter, but should be in effect for navigation of the wire through the stenosis and delivery of the dilating device. Intravenous heparin dosing can be weight-based or, better, based on activated clotting time (ACT) measurements. If weight-based, heparin can be given as an intravenous bolus of 70 to 100 units per kilogram of body weight. If ACT-based, a baseline ACT is obtained, and heparin is administered intravenously until the ACT is at least double the baseline value, or 300 to 350 seconds. Because these procedures are not usually lengthy, continuous heparin infusions after the initial dose or doses usually are not required, but if used, continuous infusions are begun at 7 to 10 units/kg/hour and adjusted by serial ACT measurements to maintain the ACT at 300 to 350 seconds.

In the special circumstance in which a IIb/IIIa platelet inhibitor is used during a procedure, either as a substitute for oral antiplatelet medication or to treat a thromboembolic complication, the heparin dosing is adjusted or partially reversed to achieve an ACT of approximately 160 seconds, to reduce the risk of a hemorrhagic complication through an additive effect of the two drugs. Administration of intravenous protamine sulfate at a dose of 10 mg for each 1000 units of heparin to be reversed is effective for this purpose, with the maximum recommended protamine dose being 80 mg. Protamine is injected slowly over 2 to 5 minutes to avoid a hypotensive reaction.

Balloon versus stent-assisted angioplasty decision

It is difficult to predict how an arterial stenosis will respond to simple balloon angioplasty alone. In some cases, a single balloon dilation will achieve an excellent result, without recoil, and with long-term stability. If the operator could depend on balloon angioplasty alone, it would be an ideal, usually simple to perform, procedure with minimal risk; there would be no need to place a stent, with all the associated potential problems related to placement of a permanent metallic foreign body in the artery, from the actual deployment process through late restenosis or thrombosis and the requirement for prolonged dual-drug antiplatelet therapy. Unfortunately, many intracranial stenoses treated by simple balloon angioplasty are minimally or incompletely dilated; recoil occurs shortly after the dilation; restenosis occurs on follow-up, leading to re-treatment with its associated complications; or, as is the case occasionally, a visible dissection flap is raised. One approach is always to perform simple balloon angioplasty of an intracranial arterial stenosis as a first step in the dilation process, evaluate the result, and either end the dilation process there if the result is satisfactory or go on to deploy a stent across the stenosis if the result of balloon dilation alone is unsatisfactory. Indeed, some stents are only deployable in this two-step process, and a two-step process is sometimes necessary just to deploy a balloon-mounted stent across a very tight stenosis that will not allow passage of a balloon-mounted stent delivery system without predilation.

One disadvantage of always performing a two-step procedure, a balloon predilation followed by stent deployment, is that an exchange wire left across the stenosis to replace the balloon angioplasty catheter with the stent delivery system can move easily during the exchange, with the tip winding up proximal to the stenosis or much further out a distal branch, where a perforation could occur. Another disadvantage of the two-step process (eg, the self-expanding Wingspan, Boston Scientific Corp., Natick, MA) is that the arterial stenosis is manipulated and dilated by devices twice rather than once, increasing the risk for rupture or a thromboembolic complication. The alternative approach, always placing a stent across the stenosis as the first step in the dilation process, has the advantage of reliable dilation of the stenosis to the desired extent (assuming the stent can be positioned and deployed) with a single manipulation of the vessel, but the disadvantages of more difficult or sometimes impossible catheter positioning and the earlier-noted issues related to the presence of an intra-arterial foreign body. No clear consensus exists on this issue. The authors' preference is to perform a single-step procedure and deploy a stent whenever the anatomy will permit, reserving balloon predilation for extremely tight stenoses.

An attempt at stent deployment may not be appropriate in certain circumstances. In cases where tortuous anatomy would preclude or potentially complicate stent placement, where the stenosed arteries to be treated are too small in diameter or too distal to be stented, or where the stenosed arterial segment is longer than any available stent of the appropriate diameter, balloon angioplasty alone may be the only desired dilation step. After assessing the stenosis and deciding the route that must be taken to reach the stenosis on the initial angiogram, and deciding whether to dilate the stenosis first with a balloon or to go straight to deployment of a stent, a device selection is made.

Dilation device selection

In order to reduce the risk of rupture of fragile intracranial arteries, a dilation generally is performed up to a diameter slightly less than that of the normal vessel segments just proximal and distal to a target stenosis. The goal most often sought is to dilate the stenosis with a balloon to about 80% of the diameter of the vessel in an adjacent, nondiseased segment, erring on the conservative side if the proximal and distal vessel diameters adjacent to the stenosis differ. A balloon angioplasty catheter is selected with a maximum diameter of 80% to 100% of the normal vessel diameter, if possible, and inflated to a point about 80% of the normal diameter. A currently available, low-profile, relatively trackable balloon angioplasty catheter with balloon sizes appropriate for intracranial arterial diameters is the Maverick (Boston Scientific Corporation), which comes in diameters of 1.5, 2.0, 2.5, 2.75, 3.0, 3.25, 3.5, 3.75, and 4.0 mm and in lengths ranging from 9 to 20 mm, depending on balloon diameters. Dual markers on most Maverick balloons indicate the proximal and distal extents of the balloon for positioning, but the 1.5-mm balloon has only a single marker to indicate the midpoint of the balloon. The balloon chosen should be of a length longer than the stenosis, but the shorter the balloon, the more easily it can be maneuvered. The Maverick is advanced over a 0.014-in guidewire and inflated to 6 to 12 atmospheres pressure. The Gateway balloon (Boston Scientific Corporation) used with the Wingspan intracranial stent system is similar to the Maverick and available in a 2.25-mm diameter, in addition to those also listed for the Maverick, and in lengths of 9, 15, and 20 mm for each diameter.

These balloon angioplasty catheters, despite being relatively trackable, are designed to treat atherosclerotic stenoses and are still stiffer than most microcatheters used for other intracranial interventions. At times, they stretch or distort intracranial arteries. If these balloons cannot be advanced into position satisfactorily, other balloons usually can be, but they are of a more compliant design and will be less likely to achieve the degree of dilation of an atherosclerotic plaque than the less-compliant balloons. A balloon catheter, such as the HyperGlide (EV3, Irvine, CA), is available in a 4.0-mm balloon diameter and 10- to 30-mm balloon lengths, and advanced over a 0.010-in guidewire, is more suitable for reversal of vasospasm than for reversal of atherosclerotic stenosis, but may be navigated to a stenosis not reachable by a Maverick or other angioplasty balloon because of its more trackable monolumen design. The dilation of an atherosclerotic stenosis achieved with such a balloon will usually be very limited because balloon size options are limited, and use of such a balloon for this purpose is limited to situations in which it is the only option.

Stent selection is more involved. The choices include balloon-mounted and self-expanding stents, bare metal and drug-eluting stents, and open-cell and closed-cell stents, with each type having various advantages and disadvantages. The first task is to choose an appropriate stent size.

Just as is the case for balloon angioplasty alone, stent-assisted angioplasty in intracranial arteries is performed more conservatively than in extracranial locations, to lower the risk for rupture of the vessel. Aiming for dilating a stenosis to 80% of the normal diameter of the vessel is quite reasonable, although one would not want to choose a stent that would not contact or be in apposition with the vessel walls proximal or distal to the stenosis because nonapposition of stent walls is believed to predispose to later thrombosis. What helps in the selection process is that a stent usually expands proximally and distally more quickly and completely than it does in its middle portion when the middle portion is centered on a stenosis, so that stent walls are apposed at the stenosis, and proximal and distal to the stenosis, despite the variability in diameter of the vessel through the treated segment. What also helps in the selection process is knowledge that a balloon-mounted stent's final deployed diameter can be varied to some extent by the maximum inflation pressure used during expansion of the balloon. In actual practice, a balloon-mounted stent usually is chosen to have a maximum diameter equal to the normal arterial diameter adjacent to the stenosis where the stent must contact the normal vessel wall. Stent diameter sizing is less critical for self-expanding stents, because delivering an oversized, self-expanding stent does not expose the vessel wall to the same force as delivering an oversized balloon-mounted stent. The length of the stent chosen is influenced somewhat by the standard lengths available for a given stent diameter, but ordinarily, it should bridge the entire focally stenotic segment and overlap slightly with the normal vessel segments proximal and distal to the stenosis, if possible. The disadvantage of choosing a stent much longer than the stenotic segment is that the longer the stent, the more difficult it will be to navigate the stent delivery system into position. In particularly tortuous anatomy, it is sometimes necessary to deliver two overlapping short stents because a single stent long enough to traverse the stenosis cannot be navigated into a satisfactory position.

Stent sizes depend on type and manufacturer. Currently, self-expanding stents are available in labeled diameters of 2.5, 3.0, 3.5, 4.0, and 4.5 mm and in lengths of 9, 15, and 20 mm. The actual maximum diameters of these stents when fully expanded are slightly greater than the labeled diameters (eg, an actual diameter of 4.4 mm for the stent labeled 4.0 mm). The manufacturer recommends using these stents in arteries in which the normal vessel diameters are from 0.5 mm smaller than the labeled stent diameter up to the same

size as the labeled stent diameters (eg, in a 3.5- to 4.0-mm vessel for a stent labeled 4.0-mm diameter). A chart is provided by the manufacturer in the product ordering information to assist in stent size selection.

Balloon-mounted stents typically are available in labeled diameters of 2.25 through 4.0 mm and in lengths that vary by manufacturer from 8 through 33 mm. For example, drug-eluting stents are available in diameters of 2.5, 2.75, 3.0, and 3.5 mm, and in lengths of 8, 13, 18, 23, 28, and 33 mm, whereas bare metal stents are available diameters of 2.25, 2.5, 2.75, 3.0, 3.5, and 4.0 mm, and in lengths of 8, 9, 12, 14, 15, 18, 24, and 30 mm. These stents can usually be dilated to diameters slightly smaller or larger than their labeled diameters according to diameter-atmosphere charts in the packaging or on the box. A 2.25-mm stent, for example, reaches a diameter of 2.25 mm at the "nominal" pressure of 6 atmospheres, and a diameter of 2.5 mm at the "rated" pressure of 16 atmospheres, with the "rated" pressure being the maximum pressure to which the balloon on the delivery catheter should be subjected, as recommended by the manufacturer. The labeled diameter of a self-expanding stent usually is chosen to be equal in diameter to the normal arterial segment adjacent to the stenosis. The ending stent diameter's dependence on the amount of pressure applied to the balloon is quite useful to compensate for any inaccuracy in preliminary vessel diameter measurements, to allow for slight undersizing in the stenotic segment, and to limit stress on the vessel walls adjacent to the stenosis.

Other characteristics of balloon-mounted stents should be considered in choosing a device. Stents can be of an open-cell design, such as the Taxus (Boston Scientific Corporation), Express II (Boston Scientific Corporation), and Driver (Medtronic) stents, or a closed-cell design, such as the Cypher (Cordis) stents. They may have thicker struts made of stainless steel (eg, Express II) or thinner struts made of a chromium alloy (eg, MicroDriver). No clear evidence indicates which cell design, strut thickness, or metal is superior in the long term, although stent structure could influence subsequent vessel wall responses, such as intimal hyperplasia and restenosis. The structure of the stent and the balloon on which the stent is mounted influence the device's flexibility, profile, and ability to cross a tight stenosis during delivery. Generally, the more flexible and narrower the profile, the easier delivery will be, as is the case with shorter stent length.

Finally, a choice must be made between bare metal and drug-eluting stents. A polymer impregnated with sirolimus, a macrocyclic lactone produced by *Streptomyces hygroscopicus,* is applied to the Cypher stent. Sirolimus inhibits smooth muscle and endothelial proliferation. A polymer containing paclitaxel, a substance originally found in the Pacific Yew tree and now synthesized to produce an anticancer drug, is applied to the Taxus stent. The Cypher stent releases almost 100% of its sirolimus over 1 month's time, whereas the second stent releases about 10% of its paclitaxel over 2 month's time, with the difference in elution rates attributed to differences in the polymer coatings.

Currently, the only devices that have been approved by the US Food and Drug Administration (FDA) for intracranial angioplasty and stenting of atherosclerotic stenosis are the Gateway balloon and the Wingspan self-expanding stent. Other devices are FDA-approved for other indications and are used "off label" for treatment of intracranial stenosis. FDA approval of the Wingspan system is through a Humanitarian Device Exemption, which requires review by an institution's human studies committee to determine whether a separate consent form will be required by the institution before clinical use in patients.

Whether a bare balloon angioplasty catheter or a balloon-mounted stent delivery catheter is selected, it should be prepared carefully for use so that air from the outer lumen connecting the balloon hub with the balloon is aspirated and replaced with a solution of contrast and saline (eg, 75% contrast). It will be important to see fluoroscopically the progress of balloon dilation in the subsequent intracranial angioplasty step, including the first parts of the balloon that expand and the full extent of balloon expansion in various arterial segments during expansion when pressure is being applied and gradually increased to the balloon. If there is no contrast in the dead space of the balloon lumen, the expansion could be much greater than appreciated fluoroscopically.

Wire selection

Most balloons and stents used intracranially for treatment of atherosclerotic stenoses are designed for introduction over 0.014-in guidewires. The ideal wire for guiding and supporting these devices would be one with a tip that could be shaped and steered easily, sturdy enough to retain its shape, yet soft enough not to dissect or perforate delicate intracranial arteries or undermine irregular plaque traversing a tight stenosis. It would also have a body or shaft that would be firm enough for a dilation device to track the course of the vessel, yet flexible enough to navigate tortuous curves without distorting the vessel and its adjacent anatomy. Because no ideal wire exists to handle every situation,

each available wire is a compromise, with certain advantages and disadvantages; however, many wires prove suitable. Most come in standard (180- to 190-cm) lengths for primary navigation of balloon or stent delivery systems and in exchange (300- to 360-cm) lengths for replacement of microcatheters used for the primary navigation through a stenosis.

The Transend EX platinum-tipped 0.014-in wire (Boston Scientific Corporation) is used commonly for many other intracranial interventions using microcatheters and is a good starting point in wire selection for intracranial atherosclerotic stenosis-dilating device navigation, fulfilling the distal flexibility and softness criteria and providing light-to-medium support proximal to its tip. The Wingspan microcatheter-delivered, self-expanding stent is designed to be used with a Transend 0.014-in wire, and the wire often proves suitable also for guiding less flexible balloon-mounted stent delivery catheters and balloon angioplasty catheters, particularly if there is relatively little vessel tortuosity proximal to the target stenosis. The platinum tip has reasonable shape retention, is not likely to perforate distal branches, is fairly steerable, and is easily seen fluoroscopically. The flexibility of this wire proximal to the tip is not likely to distort arterial curves or stretch delicate anatomy. The exchange-length version of the wire is the 300-cm floppy.

Other 0.014-in wires are currently available from various manufacturers. Abbott Vascular (formerly Guidant and now part of Boston Scientific) offers the Balance Middle Weight (BMW) wire in medium support and the Balance Heavy Weight (BHW) wire in firm support, as well as the High Torque (HT) Advance wire line. Cordis offers the SteerIt and Stabilizer lines, with the SteerIt wires allowing tip deflection adjustments from the torque device near the catheter hub. Boston Scientific also offers the ChoICE line of wires and the PT^2 line of wires in floppy to extra support versions. If a stent delivery or balloon angioplasty catheter fails to track over a light-to-medium support wire, a firmer wire can be used with the device, with the understanding that if there is relatively severe tortuosity present, the firmer wire may straighten or distort the anatomy to allow deployment of the device.

Advancement and positioning of dilation device

With the patient immobilized under general anesthesia and medicated to limit thromboembolic risks, the guide catheter positioned, the initial angiography performed, and the device selections made, road maps, preferably biplane, should be acquired in optimal working projections to define the stenosis. Ideally, the primary working projection should have enough magnification to see the lesion easily, to enable safe and efficient manipulation of the 0.014-in guidewire through and beyond the stenosis, and to permit positioning of the dilation device accurately at the stenosis, but not so much magnification that the tip of the wire is not visible distally in the arterial tree. It is important to be able to monitor the tip of the wire, which can move proximally and lessen support for the device, or move distally and dissect or perforate a branch during advancement of, or exchange for, a balloon angioplasty or stent delivery catheter. In a biplane procedure suite, the secondary working projection can be used to monitor the wire tip position, if a more magnified view on the primary working projection is desirable for treatment of the stenosis. At least one road-mapped working projection should display the stenosis and the arterial segments proximal and distal to the stenosis as close to perpendicular to the line between the image intensifier and tube as possible, with little to no overlap or telescoping of the vessel, so that balloon or stent positioning will be correct.

With the balloon angioplasty or stent delivery system prepared, air aspirated and purged from the entire system, the wire preshaped to navigate through the artery to the stenotic segment, and rotating hemostatic valves placed at the hub of the guide catheter and at the hub or hubs of the balloon angioplasty or stent delivery catheter and connected to regulated pressurized infusions of heparinized saline, the device chosen for initial dilation, or, in the case of an intended exchange procedure, the microcatheter, is introduced through the guide catheter into the internal carotid or vertebral artery selected, then advanced over the wire until the wire is in a position just proximal to the target stenosis and just distal to the distal marker of the device.

At this point, it is good to stop and reassess the patient and the planned procedure. What is the systemic arterial blood pressure? Is it at a desirable level? If not, the anesthesiologist should adjust it, and be prepared to readjust it, if necessary, during or after the dilation. Is the patient fully anesthetized and immobilized? If not, that fundamental requirement should be addressed before attempting the dilation. A patient awakening or moving during what should be a slow, gentle dilation of a balloon or a precise deployment of a stent in a delicate intracranial artery raises the risk for an arterial injury or an undesirable result. Has there been any distortion of the arterial anatomy as a result of the advancement of the wire and device to this point since the original road maps were acquired, or have the road maps become degraded for any

reason? If so, the road maps should be repeated. One should be sure that when the wire is advanced in the next step, it is in the intended path, directed through the stenosis and along a defined arterial tree. Now that the balloon or stent markers are in the same field of view as the stenosis on the screen, are there any surprises about their lengths? If the device appears too short to do the job or so long that it potentially would injure other branches, now would be the time to select a different device. Finally, is the shape of the wire tip correct to traverse the stenosis, now that it has navigated the artery to a point just proximal to the stenosis? If not, it should be removed, reshaped, and reintroduced through the rotating hemostatic valve.

The wire is then advanced as atraumatically as possible through the target stenosis. Sometimes a wire needs to be exchanged for a wire with different characteristics, such as a more easily shaped, softer, or more easily torqued tip, to traverse a given stenosis. For example, a Syncho 0.014-in wire (Boston Scientific Corporation) with a softer, more easily torqued tip, or an Agility 0.014-in wire (Cordis) with a tip that can be shaped more acutely with good shape retention, may perform better than an initially selected general-use wire in traversing a stenosis, though offering less support for device advancement in the case of the Synchro, or less tip softness in the case of the Agility. Once the wire is guided successfully through the stenosis, the tip is advanced further distally in the arterial tree, well beyond the stenosis, if possible. The further out the arterial tree the wire is advanced beyond the stenosis, the better support the dilation device will have for advancement into its final position, but the wire tip should not be so far out that it does not still move freely within the artery without the constraint of too small a distal arterial diameter or too great an angulation of a small distal branch, to avoid the possibility of perforation. If the first step was to deliver the wire with a microcatheter and exchange for the dilation device, the microcatheter is removed over the exchange-length wire and replaced with the dilation device at this point, taking care to observe and maintain a stable position of the wire tip during the exchange.

With the wire tip in position distal to the stenosis and road maps without misregistration, the balloon or stent is advanced until its markers are positioned across the target stenosis. In some cases, a stenosis is so tight that passage of a selected dilation system is not possible. Resistance is encountered, which may result in kinking or looping of the balloon catheter or stent delivery system, retrograde displacement of the guiding catheter, or undue force being exerted on the artery at the site of stenosis. If such resistance is encountered, the stenosis probably needs to be predilated with a smaller-diameter, lower-profile device, the smallest of which would currently be a 1.5-mm Maverick or Gateway balloon. If a predilation step is needed, it is best to do that with an exchange-length wire across the stenosis because the 1.5-mm balloon will probably need to be replaced with a larger balloon or a stent delivery system for further dilation after the predilation. It is a good idea to recheck the position of the guiding catheter and adjust it, if needed, after any additional force is applied to advance a dilation system to counter resistance, before attempting to deploy a new device, and to reset the road maps in working projections whenever a device is replaced. Sometimes a guide catheter is not stable enough to support delivery of a dilation device, particularly if resistance is encountered in advancing a system around tortuous anatomy. In such a case, if not anticipated in advance, the intracranial wire and dilation system will have to be removed and the guide catheter replaced or reinforced, as discussed earlier in the guide catheter section; then the above steps are repeated to place the wire and dilation device in proper position for treatment.

Once the balloon or stent delivery system has been advanced successfully across the target stenosis, the catheter should be adjusted so that the proximal and distal markers are in the correct positions to achieve dilation of the desired segment of the vessel. If there is any question about the final position, an angiographic run (preferably performed with a hand injection of contrast through the guiding catheter or a very gentle mechanical injection so as not to shift the position of the device) can be performed to confirm positioning, assuming the device is not occlusive within the stenosis, and assuming the angiographic equipment can image an angiographic run without loss of the road maps.

Dilation

The initial step in reversing an intracranial arterial stenosis is a balloon dilation, whether with a bare balloon angioplasty catheter or with a balloon-mounted stent delivery catheter. Once the markers for the balloon or balloon-mounted stent are aligned on each side of the stenosis, pressure to the balloon is applied using an inflation device having a calibrated pressure gauge filled with the desired contrast/saline solution. The pressure is increased gradually while the pressure readings on the inflation device gauge and the response of the balloon on the angiography monitor are observed. As emphasized earlier in the discussion about balloon and stent size selection, it is safer to underdilate than to dilate fully a fragile intracranial artery, and it is safer to dilate very gradually rather than

quickly an intracranial stenosis. Intracranial arterial rupture is a potentially devastating complication. The goal of treating an intracranial stenosis is to achieve an acceptable and adequate functional result at the lowest risk, rather than an ideal angiographic posttreatment image. As recommended by John J. (Buddy) Connors and Joan Wojak on the basis of their early extensive experience in this area, balloon inflation rates should be slow and gentle, with inflation reaching the desired diameter over the course of 2 to 5 minutes (eg, increasing pressure by 1 atmosphere every 15 seconds, once contrast is seen within the balloon, until the desired result is achieved), and with the target diameter being 80% to 100% of the normal vessel diameter, preferably a slightly undersized diameter, and never larger than the normal vessel diameter. For balloon-mounted stents, a pressure-diameter table is provided with each device so that final diameters reached can be gauged by pressures applied during inflation, but direct observation is also important during the course of inflation, to be certain that the balloon or stent diameters do not exceed normal vessel diameters on the basis of the road-mapped images. Although slight undersizing of a final stent diameter may be the desired end result, too much undersizing of a final stent diameter, such that stent margins are not apposed to the arterial walls in the normal vessel segments, is undesirable because stent margins not in contact with vessel walls can predispose to later thrombosis. The target stent diameter should be one that will not be so great as to stress the vessel wall and risk rupture, but not so small as to leave stent margins free and risk thromboembolic complications.

At times, until a bare balloon is large enough that friction between the balloon and arterial walls maintains the balloon in a stable condition, the balloon, during the initial stages of inflation, may move distally or proximally because of a "watermelon seed" phenomenon or as a result of propulsion by arterial flow. If this movement occurs, the balloon can be deflated partially or fully and moved back into position by gentle traction on, or advancement of, the balloon catheter; if necessary, gentle traction or forward force can be applied to the balloon angioplasty catheter during reinflation of the balloon to keep it stable and in position at the site of stenosis. Instability is less likely to occur during inflation of a balloon-mounted stent because a stent tends to expand at each end initially in the nonstenotic or less stenotic portions of the vessel, anchoring its position to the vessel walls. Once a stent is partially expanded, it is usually better to continue its expansion and deployment rather than attempt to reposition it partially expanded, to avoid injury to the artery, even if deployment of a second stent becomes necessary to treat a remaining segment of stenosis.

Once the desired diameter is reached, the balloon is deflated slowly and methodically until it is no longer exerting force on the arterial walls or stenotic plaque, and then fully deflated. With the wire maintained in position across the stenosis to ensure that a balloon or stent delivery system can be advanced easily and quickly back through the stenotic segment if need be, the balloon is withdrawn to a point just proximal to the stenosis to allow free contrast passage through the stenosis.

Assessment

After the initial dilation, an angiogram is performed to assess the result. This procedure can be done with a mechanical contrast injection of the guide catheter in the magnified working projections used for positioning of the device, as long as the balloon is fully deflated and retracted from the stenosis so that imaging resolution is optimal. The result is compared with the predilation images to determine the degree of residual stenosis, whether a dissection flap is visible, whether flow is at an improved or normal rate beyond the stenosis, and whether any branch or branches arising at the stenotic segment have been affected adversely by the dilation. Distal branches should also be examined for evidence of emboli.

The patient should also be reassessed at this time. A significant rise in systemic blood pressure and a decline in the pulse rate could be an indication that an arterial rupture or intracranial hemorrhage has occurred. The postdilation angiogram should be re-examined for any evidence of mass effect, shift, or general slowing of circulation time to suggest increased intracranial pressure. If hemorrhage is a valid concern, prompt reversal of the heparin with protamine is probably warranted, and an emergent CT scan of the brain should probably be obtained before further steps are taken, with removal of the balloon catheter and wire to permit the scan to be done. On the other hand, systemic blood pressure may have declined after correction of the stenosis, from a baseline elevated level to a normal level, a change that need not be compensated for, assuming flow is good through the dilated stenosis. If flow has improved significantly beyond the dilated stenosis in a hypertensive patient who has a recent or subacute infarction in the territory beyond the stenosis, it may be wise to have the anesthesiologist lower the pressure into a normotensive range rather than maintain it in a significantly elevated range, because autoregulation may be impaired and postreperfusion hemorrhage into the infarcted territory could occur with exposure to excessive pressure.

Further dilation

The operator must decide, on the basis of the patient's clinical presentation, the goals of the procedure, and the angiographic findings after the initial dilation, whether to dilate the stenosis further or accept the initial result (Fig. 3). A slight increase in linear diameter at a stenosis results in a much greater increase in flow because of the increase in cross-sectional area at the stenosis, and an initial dilation can be followed by remodeling and smoothing of a stenotic lesion over time; therefore, some operators advocate accepting even significant degrees of residual stenosis after angioplasty, as long as a measurable improvement is seen after an initial dilation. The advantage of this approach is that the risk of dilating the stenosis is minimized because manipulation of, and stress on, the vessel is minimized. The disadvantage of leaving a significant residual stenosis is that the stenosis is more likely to recur and potentially require re-treatment later, particularly in a diabetic patient. This scenario may be the best one in a patient being treated with a subacute infarction in the territory distal to the target stenosis, when a later redilation in a more elective setting might have a greater safety margin. Certainly, if the initial dilation with a balloon alone yields a result that reverses a stenosis to 20% or less, one would have to question whether the additional risk associated with placement of a stent at the sight of that stenosis is justified. Likewise, a residual stenosis of 20% or less achieved by placement of a balloon-mounted stent would be quite satisfactory, and a desirable end result, in most cases. Even 40% or less residual stenosis after initial dilation would be judged by many to be evidence that the goal of treatment had been achieved, assuming, if a stent had been placed, that the stent margins contacted vessel walls on both sides of the stenosis.

If, after the initial dilation, residual stenosis is significant, the dilation was with a balloon-mounted stent, and the residual narrowing is within the stented portion of the vessel, the balloon can be advanced over the wire back to the waist in the stenotic segment and dilated to a larger diameter, if the initial dilation was too conservative. Again, care should be taken not to overdilate the vessel and to dilate the stenosis slowly. If the residual stenosis is in a segment of the artery that is beyond the margins of the initially placed stent, redilating with the balloon can also be attempted, but it may be necessary to place a second stent at the site of residual stenosis, particularly if the initial stent was not aligned optimally across the stenosis or if the initial stent proved to be too short to cover the entire length of the plaque. If no stent was placed, the initial dilation was performed with a bare balloon, and residual stenosis is significant after the initial balloon dilation, as is often the case, a stent can be deployed across the stenosis. In that case, the balloon angioplasty catheter must be withdrawn over the exchange-length wire and replaced with a stent delivery catheter, again taking care to observe the behavior of the tip of the wire during the exchange. The stent can be self-expanding, such as the Wingspan, or balloon-mounted. In general, the additional expansion of the vessel at the site of residual stenosis after a bare balloon dilation will be more limited with a self-expanding stent than with a balloon-mounted stent. The choice between the two types of stents will factor in the degree of residual stenosis, the tortuosity of the anatomy, and the size of the vessel. A greater degree of residual stenosis, a larger, more proximal vessel segment, and a straighter course to navigate with the delivery device would tend to favor selection of a balloon-mounted stent, whereas tortuous anatomy, a lesser degree of residual stenosis, and a more fragile vessel segment would tend to favor selection of a self-expanding, microcatheter-delivered stent.

The steps taken for delivery and deployment of a balloon-mounted stent are as described earlier for the initial angioplasty. The steps taken for deployment of a Wingspan stent are different. This stent is packaged sandwiched between an inner and outer microcatheter. The coaxial microcatheter system (an outer catheter and an inner stabilizer catheter) is advanced over the wire to the stenosis, the stent markers are positioned proximal and distal to the stenosis, usually into the adjacent normal vessel segments, the system is retracted to eliminate redundancy or coils and to straighten the catheter system as much as possible without moving the stent markers, and then the stent is deployed by fixing the inner stabilizer catheter and withdrawing the outer catheter, allowing the stent to expand from distally to proximally as it is uncovered. The catheter system is then removed over the wire. (Further information about deploying this device can be found in its instructions for use, provided by the manufacturer.)

Just as for the initial dilation, any further dilation should be followed by an assessment of the patient's clinical and angiographic response to the intervention. Ordinarily, any second dilation performed corrects or improves the appearance of the target stenosis. If a second balloon-mounted stent has been deployed across a segment of stenosis not treated by the first deployed stent, and residual stenosis is significant within that second stent, it can be dilated further with the balloon, as described earlier. If there is still residual stenosis following deployment of the Wingspan stent, no further steps

are generally taken at the time of the initial treatment session, unless a complication needs to be addressed.

Complications

One serious complication of the procedure can be arterial rupture, leading to subarachnoid hemorrhage and interference with flow into the artery distal to the site of injury. One measure to limit arterial bleeding is immediate reversal of systemic heparin anticoagulation with intravenous protamine sulfate (10 mg of protamine sulfate per 1000 units of heparin to be reversed, up to a maximum dose of 80 mg). If contrast extravasation is still seen, gentle inflation of a balloon, often one already in the artery, in a position proximal to the stenosis and site of injury, just sufficient to occlude flow temporarily, can be performed to limit bleeding further. Reversing the effects of antiplatelet drugs, obtaining and transfusing platelets, takes time, and bleeding is often stopped by the time platelets are available. One unfortunate result of reversal of anticoagulation and antiplatelet drugs may be thrombosis of the arterial segment at the site of angioplasty or stent deployment, resulting in distal cerebral infarction. Rupture of the vessel can increase intracranial pressure and be fatal, but measures to lower intracranial pressure with drugs such as intravenous mannitol must be taken cautiously because cerebral perfusion pressure (the intracranial pressure subtracted from the mean systemic arterial pressure) must be maintained at about 50 to 60 mm Hg to maintain viability. Fortunately, arterial rupture is rare when the earlier dilation guidelines are followed. It is a complication much better avoided than treated to achieve a good clinical end result.

Another complication of the procedure can be a visible dissection, either at the site of angioplasty or elsewhere in the arterial tree, as a result of manipulation by catheters, wires, or dilation devices. If the dissection is at the site of stenosis after a simple bare balloon angioplasty or elsewhere in the arterial tree, flow is normal, there is no significant residual stenosis, and no significant thrombus has formed, the decision can be made simply to continue the heparin infusion overnight, continue the antiplatelet drugs, and re-examine the stenosis angiographically the day after the procedure. At that point, if the appearance is stable or improving, the heparin can be discontinued, the antiplatelet drugs continued, and the dissection allowed to heal and remodel. If, however, the dissection at the time of the balloon dilation is seen to interfere with flow, it would probably be best to deploy a stent across the stenosis and dissection, leaving an exchange-length wire across

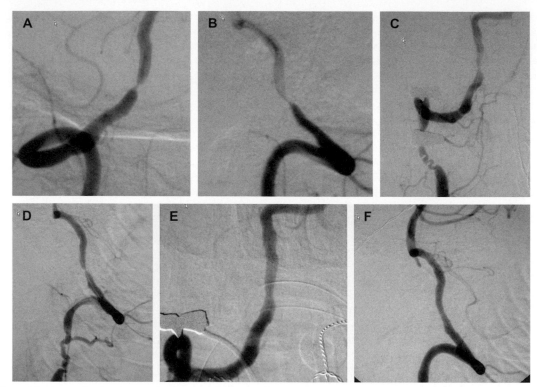

Fig. 3. Distal vertebral artery angioplasty and stenting for a symptomatic stenosis. This patient was a 56-year-old man with a recent pontine stroke. He was placed on warfarin after MR angiography demonstrated bilateral distal vertebral artery stenoses. He had two TIAs on warfarin and was referred for angioplasty and stenting. Initial posteroanterior (*A*) and lateral (*B*) projections of the right vertebral artery stenosis. A 6F guide catheter was placed in the proximal right vertebral artery from a femoral approach. A 300 cm 0.014 in wire was placed across the stenosis. A 2.5 mm × 8 mm balloon-expandable stent would not cross the stenosis. The standard wire was replaced with another 300 cm 0.014 in wire with greater support, and the stent was deployed. Posteroanterior (*C*) and lateral (*D*) projections showing residual stenosis and telescoping and vasospasm of the vertebral artery proximal to the stenosis. The 300 cm wire was removed. A 2.5 mm × 10 mm balloon was placed primarily aross the stenosis over a standard 0.014 in wire for a repeat dilation. Final posteroanterior (*E*) and lateral (*F*) projections showing minimal residual stenosis and resolution of the wire-induced vasospasm.

the lesion and following the earlier steps to place a self-expanding or balloon-mounted stent. If the dissection has led to significant thrombus formation and the thrombus is interfering with flow or may potentially fragment and migrate with placement of a stent, it would probably be best to accelerate lysis of the clot before further intervention, either with intravenous abciximab (an initial 0.20 mg/kg intravenous bolus, followed by a continuous infusion of 0.125 ug/kg/min, up to a maximum infusion rate of 10 ug/kg/min for up to 12 hours) or with a fibrinolytic drug administered intra-arterially at the site of the clot by way of a microcatheter. Use of intravenous abciximab or an intra-arterial fibrinolytic drug increases the risk for a hemorrhagic complication, and reducing the ACT to 160 seconds or less with intravenous protamine sulfate, if needed to reverse the heparin effect partially before administration of those additional drugs, is recommended.

Embolism distal to the treated stenosis is another potential complication of treatment. The degree of obstruction caused by the embolus or emboli, whether the affected territory is eloquent or noneloquent, and the degree to which collateral flow compensates for the embolism all influence whether specific intervention is indicated for this complication, beyond continuing heparin anticoagulation and oral antiplatelet drugs. Minor emboli in noneloquent territories or with good pial collateral flow distal to the emboli often are not treated with additional interventions. Lysis of major distal emboli can be performed under the earlier guidelines with intravenous abciximab or a microcatheter-delivered intra-arterial fibrinolytic drug.

It would be reasonable to perform a postprocedure, noncontrast brain CT scan immediately after the procedure in a case in which a fibrinolytic drug has been given or an additional intervention has been performed, to be certain there is no angiographically unsuspected hemorrhage or to document the extent of angiographically suspected subarachnoid, intraventricular, or intraparenchymal hemorrhage. Unsuspected hemorrhages found on CT scanning may influence the choice of drugs given in the postprocedure period or prompt other interventions, such as ventriculostomy.

Just as in other interventions, minor technical complications or issues can arise during intracranial angioplasty or stent placement. Vasospasm can be induced in cervical or intracranial arteries from catheter or wire manipulation or advancement or withdrawal of devices. Most often, a time delay will result in sufficient relaxation of vasospasm, but intra-arterial administration of papaverine (eg, 3 mg/mL in normal saline for a total dose of 30 to 100 mg, depending on response, delivered slowly over 15 to 60 minutes to avoid increasing intracranial pressure) or verapamil (eg, 1 mg/mL in normal saline for a total dose of 3 to 10 mg, depending on effect, delivered over 3 to 10 minutes to avoid systemic hypotension) can hasten vessel relaxation.

Postprocedure management

Just as systemic blood pressure management is important to observe and manage during the case, it is also important following a successful dilation, particularly in the patient who has subacute infarction in the territory distal to the treated stenosis. Hypertension should be corrected to reduce the risk for perfusion pressure breakthrough bleeding in the infarcted territory. Blood pressure most often can be brought back into a normal range in patients in whom it was allowed to rise to help perfuse ischemic territory beyond a stenosis.

Most often, heparin is discontinued immediately following the procedure. If there is excellent flow, a smoothly reversed stenosis, no thrombus, and a subacute infarction in the territory distal to the angioplastied or stented arterial segment, immediate reversal of the heparin with intravenous protamine can be performed at the conclusion of the case. Likewise, if the result of dilation is good and the sheath must be removed from the arterial access site immediately, heparin can be reversed for its removal.

Heparin therapy can be continued until the next day or longer if there is thrombus or significant luminal irregularity to predispose to thrombus formation following dilation. In such a case, the heparin infusion can be adjusted to maintain the partial thromboplastin time in a desirable range (eg, 50–80 seconds).

After the patient is awakened from general anesthesia, extubated, and observed until awake and stable in the postanesthesia recovery unit, he/she is optimally placed in a neurology or neurosurgery intensive care unit for postprocedure monitoring and care overnight. Changes in neurologic status or vital signs that are concerning for thromboembolic or hemorrhagic complication can be identified and acted on early with close nursing observation. Most patients can be discharged from the hospital on the day after the procedure if recovery is uneventful.

Antiplatelet drugs are continued. Aspirin (81–325 mg daily) is usually given to all nonallergic patients on a permanent basis following intracranial angioplasty or stenting. Usually, clopidogrel (75 mg daily) is also given in combination with the aspirin for a limited time after the procedure, ranging from 30 days to a year, depending on the situation. Following balloon angioplasty alone, 30 days of clopidogrel is usually sufficient, whereas 60 days is usually sufficient after placement of a bare metal stent. The current duration of clopidogrel therapy recommended by the FDA following placement of a drug-eluting stent is 6 months. These times for dual antiplatelet drug therapy are recommended with the assumption that the patient is not having recurrent symptoms related to the stenosis, or bleeding complications related to combined drug therapy. The duration of clopidogrel therapy can be shortened if bleeding complications demand it, or lengthened if recurrent symptoms develop.

Follow-up

After discharge from the hospital, patients are followed clinically to detect any recurrent ischemic symptoms, and by reimaging the treated arterial segment to detect recurrent or in-stent stenosis. Although CT angiography and MR angiography may yield images in patients who underwent angioplasty alone with adequate resolution to exclude recurrent disease, noninvasive imaging of a stented intracranial lesion is often unsatisfactory. The best reimaging is by conventional angiography, and the follow-up examination can be limited in scope. If a patient remains asymptomatic in the postprocedure period, repeat angiography can be performed in a 3- to 6-month time frame after treatment, on the shorter end if angioplasty alone or a bare metal stent was used or if there was suboptimal reversal of the original stenosis, and on the longer end if a drug-eluting stent was used and the reversal of the original stenosis was good.

Re-treatment

If a patient has recurrent symptoms and recurrent stenosis on repeat imaging, re-treatment of the stenosis is appropriate. How the lesion should be retreated depends, in part, on how the lesion was

treated the first time, but if the patient has reste-
nosed, doing something more to reduce the risk
for recurrent stenosis could be justified. If angioplasty alone was performed and the stenosis re-
curred, placement of a stent at the recurrent
stenosis is probably the best approach. If a bare-
metal stent was placed the first time, re-treatment
with a drug-eluting stent deployed within the bare-
metal stent is a reasonable option. If a drug-eluting
stent was placed the first time and the patient developed recurrent stenosis in that stent, it is not clear
that placing another drug-eluting stent within that
stent would be any better than simply performing
a balloon angioplasty within the original drug-eluting stent, although either technique could be tried.
With re-treatment, the same precautions apply, including avoidance of overdilation of the artery.

If a patient has no recurrent symptoms, but has
recurrent stenosis at the treated lesion on follow-
up imaging, the decision to re-treat the stenosis is
more difficult and depends to some degree how
critical the restenosis is and whether collateral
flow is sufficient to support the involved territory
should the artery go on to further stenosis or occlusion. One would want to re-treat a significant recurrent stenosis if the artery were the sole supply to the
distal territory, without circle of Willis or other
compensatory flow available, but if collateral flow
were adequate and the patient asymptomatic,
continued observation would probably be the
lowest-risk approach. If the patient has recurrent
symptoms and no significant recurrent stenosis,
then continued, or more aggressive, drug treatment
would be preferred over redilation.

Summary

Dilation of stenoses of the major intracranial
arteries is now technically possible in many cases.

Device development for intracranial arterial
angioplasty and stenting will likely yield more
flexible and navigable delivery systems and new
stent designs that further lower restenosis rates.
Using proper precautions, most procedures can
be performed without complications today, but
the safety margin will likely be improved with refinement of current devices and the introduction
of new devices made specifically for this indication. Clinical efficacy is still under study and is
addressed specifically elsewhere in this publication, but early experience with these techniques
is promising for lowering the risk for recurrent ischemic events in patients who have symptomatic
intracranial arterial stenosis refractory to medical
therapy.

Further readings

Connors JJ 3rd, Wojac JC. Percutaneous transluminal
angioplasty for intracranial atherosclerotic lesions:
evolution of technique and short-term results. J
Neurosurg 1999;91:415–23.

Henkes H, Miloslavski E, Lowens S, et al. Treatment of
intracranial stenoses with balloon dilatation and
self-expanding stent deployment (Wingspan). Neuroradiology 2005;47:222–8.

Meyers PM, Higashida RT, Phatouros CC, et al. Cerebral hyperperfusion syndrome after percutaneous
transluminal stenting of the craniocervical arteries.
Neurosurgery 2000;47:335–43.

Mori T, Fukuoka M, Kazita M, et al. Follow-up study
after intracranial percutaneous transluminal angioplasty. AJNR Am J Neuroradiol 1998;19:1525–33.

Schumacher HC, Khaw AV, Meyers PM, et al. Intracranial angioplasty and stent placement for cerebral atherosclerosis. J Vasc Interv Radiol 2004;15:S123–32.

Wojak JC, Dunlap DC, Hargrave KR, et al. Intracranial
angioplasty and stenting: long-term results from a single center. AJNR Am J Neuroradiol 2006;27:1882–92.

ELSEVIER
SAUNDERS

NEUROIMAGING
CLINICS
OF NORTH AMERICA

Neuroimag Clin N Am 17 (2007) 381–392

Endovascular Treatment of Vertebral Artery–Origin and Innominate/Subclavian Disease: Indications and Technique

Guilherme Dabus, MD[a],*, Christopher J. Moran, MD[b,c],
Colin P. Derdeyn, MD[b,c,d], DeWitte T. Cross, III MD[b,c]

- Anatomy
- Mechanism and clinical presentation
- Diagnostic work-up
- Indications
- Technical aspects
- Discussion and long-term results
- Considerations for endovascular treatment of the innominate and subclavian arteries
  - *Clinical aspects*
  - *Indications for treatment*
  - *Technical aspects and results*
- References

Extracranial vertebral artery (VA) atherosclerotic disease most frequently involves the origin of the vessel. The prevalence of VA-origin stenosis varies from approximately 20% to 40% of patients who have cerebrovascular disease [1–11]. Atherosclerotic lesions of VA origin are a potential cause of posterior circulation ischemia, which can be disabling, or even deadly. Of patients experiencing posterior circulation transient ischemic attack (TIA), 22% to 35% will suffer an infarct within 5 years of the TIA, with a mortality rate of 20% to 30%

[4,11,12]. Patients who have atherosclerotic disease of VA origin are treated initially with antiplatelet medications or anticoagulation. A high degree of stenosis (greater than 50%) or failure of medical therapy prompts intervention, either open surgery or endovascular procedures. Surgery usually is successful technically; however, it is also associated with high rates of procedural and periprocedural complications [7,8,11,13]. For these reasons, new techniques and technologies that can be used in the treatment of such lesions are being developed.

[a] Division of Interventional Neuroradiology, Gray 241, Massachusetts General Hospital – Harvard Medical School, 55 Fruit Street, Boston, MA 02114, USA
[b] Division of Interventional Neuroradiology, Mallinckrodt Institute of Radiology – Washington University School of Medicine, 510 South Kingshighway, St. Louis, MO 63110, USA
[c] Department of Neurological Surgery, Washington University School of Medicine, 510 South Kingshighway, St. Louis, MO 63110, USA
[d] Department of Neurology, Washington University School of Medicine, 510 South Kingshighway, St. Louis, MO 63110, USA
* Corresponding author.
E-mail address: gdabus@partners.org (G. Dabus).

doi:10.1016/j.nic.2007.03.005

Since the 1990s, percutaneous angioplasty and stenting have gained increasing importance as the first treatment modality for this patient population. Angioplasty and stenting of the VA origin, although technically simple, can be challenging, depending on the anatomic features of the aortic arch, brachiocephalic trunk, and subclavian arteries. Despite possible technical challenges, multiple clinical series and case reports have been published in the medical literature showing the feasibility, safety, and efficacy of this procedure in the treatment of symptomatic atherosclerotic lesions of VA origin [4–8,10–22].

Anatomy

The left VA frequently is larger than the right VA. The anatomy of the extracranial VA varies little between individuals. Usually, the VA is the first and largest branch of the subclavian artery, originating from its superior-posterior wall [11,23]. The left VA arising directly from the aortic arch between the left common carotid artery and the left subclavian artery, rather than from the subclavian artery, is the most common variation (2%–5%). Beyond its origin, the VA runs behind the anterior scalenus muscle with a cephalad, slightly posterior trajectory, entering the foramina transversarium of C6 in 88% of people, C5 or C7 in 6% of people, and C4 in 4% of people [23].

The VA is divided into four segments. The first segment (V1) extends from its origin to its entrance into the foramina transversaria. The second segment (V2) extends from its entrance into the foramina transversaria to C2, and ascends almost straight, passing through the foramina transversarium of each vertebra to C2. As patients age, this segment can become tortuous and can be impinged on by bony spurs arising from the cervical spine. The third segment (V3) extends from C2 to the point at which the VA pierces the dura mater. Within this segment, the VA leaves the foramina transversarium of C2, forming a lateral convex curve, reaching the foramen of C1, and then running backward and subsequently antero-superiorly. The fourth segment (V4), also known as the intradural segment, extends from the point at which the VA enters the dura mater to the vertebrobasilar junction [11,23]. Muscular branches originate from the second and third segments of the VA, supplying the cervical muscles with rich anastomoses to the thyrocervical and costocervical trunks and the external carotid artery [11]. The knowledge of these anastomoses is extremely important because these anastomoses can provide an important collateral source for reconstitution of the distal VA in instances of severe proximal atherosclerotic disease.

Description and discussion of the rare anatomic variations of the subclavian and VA is beyond the scope of this article. The reader, however, should learn the possible locations of the subclavian and VA origins from imaging of the patient, including arch aortography.

Mechanism and clinical presentation

Vertebrobasilar insufficiency is an underdiagnosed clinical condition and usually is associated with nonspecific symptoms (such as dizziness) that also may be caused by other arterial territories [2,5,7].

Different mechanisms can cause symptoms of vertebrobasilar ischemia in the setting of extracranial VA stenosis, including artery-to-artery embolism and hemodynamic impairment when associated with stenosis, occlusion, hypoplasia, or absence of the contralateral VA [1–11]. Another factor that needs to be considered is the characteristic of the VA-origin plaque. VA-origin plaque tends to be hard, smooth, concentric, and less prone to ulceration or intramural hemorrhage and, therefore, carries less risk of embolism, compared with carotid bifurcation plaque [1,4,6,12]. Nevertheless, the proximal extracranial VA disease in the New England Medical Center Posterior Circulation Registry, where data from 407 consecutive patients were evaluated, revealed that 20% of these patients had lesions in the V1 segment of the VA. The analysis of these data demonstrated that the cause of posterior circulation ischemic events was artery-to-artery embolism from VA origin in 24% of the population studied, and that this number increased to almost 50% when possible artery-to-artery embolism cases were added [2]. The same study also showed that hemodynamic TIA due to bilateral vertebral disease was a less common, but significant, mechanism, accounting for 16% of the study population [2].

Embolism usually affects the distal circulation with a sudden onset of maximal neurologic symptoms and signs, which may resolve spontaneously (TIA). An infarct with an embolic source is more likely to result in parenchymal hemorrhage than an infarct with a hemodynamic cause [11]. Some investigators state that hemodynamic impairment is the most important mechanism of infarct formation when embolic cardiac sources are excluded [7,9,10]. Hemodynamic symptoms usually result from stenosis when associated with occlusion, hypoplasia, absence, or severe stenosis of the contralateral VA, limiting the blood flow to the parenchyma in the vertebrobasilar distribution. The resulting decrease in perfusion and the degree of collateral circulation determine the occurrence of symptoms. Even asymptomatic patients can become symptomatic if the arterial blood pressure is decreased, thereby decreasing the parenchymal perfusion [11].

Multiple symptoms have been associated with atherosclerotic disease of VA origin resulting in vertebrobasilar ischemia, including posterior circulation strokes and persistent symptoms of vertebrobasilar insufficiency. Dizziness, vertigo, impaired balance, dysarthria, syncope, diplopia, ataxia, nausea, vomiting, tinnitus, cortical blindness and visual deficit, memory disturbance, nystagmus, motor or sensory complaints, facial palsy and numbness, dysphagia, mental status changes, and decreased level of consciousness are all symptoms and signs that may be related to vertebrobasilar ischemia [7,11].

Diagnostic work-up

The VA origin is a segment difficult to image [2,5,7,10]. Color Doppler ultrasound may offer good views, providing important diagnostic and hemodynamic information [8]. Developments in the protocols of imaging modalities such as CT angiography and MR angiography are improving the visualization of the VA origin, allowing faster diagnosis of VA-origin disease. Catheter angiography remains the gold standard for quantification of the degree of stenosis at the VA origin, evaluation of the plaque, detection of ulceration or thrombus, and assessment of the extra- and intracranial collateral circulation. A complete four-vessel study is essential to evaluate possible lesions in the carotid arteries, subclavian arteries, and intracranial vessels; it also identifies VA dominance and gives important clues regarding the mechanism of vertebrobasilar ischemia (embolic versus hemodynamic).

A cross-sectional study of the brain parenchyma with CT, or preferably MR imaging, should be performed to assess for acute or old infarcts, ischemia, or hemorrhage, because these findings will have a major impact in the decision-making process.

Indications

Classically, vertebrobasilar insufficiency is treated initially with antiplatelet agents, anticoagulants, or a combination of both (see Refs. [5,7,11,13,14]). Medical treatment regimens for vertebrobasilar insufficiency are derived from carotid studies' data; unfortunately, it is not clear if medical therapy has any benefit or if it should be the first line of treatment [6]. When optimal medical therapy fails to prevent posterior circulation ischemic symptoms, endovascular techniques can be proposed. The reason is that, in these selected cases, the potential benefits of the endovascular treatment (angioplasty and stenting) outweigh the risks of the procedure.

At our institution, patients presenting with posterior circulation ischemic symptoms despite optimal medical therapy, and who have a digital subtraction angiogram demonstrating VA-origin stenosis greater than 50%, are considered for endovascular therapy.

If the source of posterior circulation ischemic events is thought to be embolic and no other sources of arterial embolism are found (cardiac), it is reasonable to assume that the symptoms are the result of artery-to-artery embolism from the diseased VA origin. For this reason, even if the stenosis is less then 50%, we believe that it should be considered for treatment because it may be the source of embolism. The neointima that develops following angioplasty and stenting may protect against future distal embolism by smoothing luminal irregularities, thereby decreasing flow turbulence at the origin of the vessel [7,12,14].

The treatment of asymptomatic patients who have significant stenosis of VA origin is a subject of controversy. Although most asymptomatic patients do not require endovascular treatment, some investigators believe that high-grade stenosis (greater then 70%) affecting the origin of a dominant or single VA should be treated because of a possible increased risk of stroke [11]. Other investigators believe asymptomatic patients should be treated when the necessity of collateral support is of major importance (as in cases of carotid occlusion) [7]. VA stenosis may become symptomatic when hypertensive patients, or even normotensive patients, have a reduction in their blood pressure.

Technical aspects

All patients should have a complete history elicited and a neurologic examination for intra- and postprocedure comparison. A complete cervicocranial angiogram should be performed to evaluate the target lesion, the collateral pathways, the direction of flow, and the presence of asymptomatic stenosis that could influence the decision process for the procedure.

As per our protocol, all elective patients are pretreated for 5 days with clopidogrel bisulfate 75 mg per day, in addition to aspirin, 325 mg per day. The antiplatelet pretreatment regimen is extremely important to decrease the risk of stent thrombosis after endothelial injury, or plaque rupture following angioplasty and stenting [11]. In urgent cases, patients can be loaded with 300 mg of clopidogrel bisulfate in addition to aspirin on the day of the procedure. Another option is a bolus infusion of glycoprotein IIb/IIIa inhibitors concomitantly with a loading dose of oral antiplatelet agents just before the procedure.

An interesting procedural point is the use of conscious sedation versus general anesthesia. Most of our procedures are performed using local anesthesia and conscious sedation, which allows serial neurologic examinations throughout the procedure, enabling recognition of procedural complications and hastening their treatment. We reserve general anesthesia for patients for whom problems with airway control or patient motion are anticipated.

The arterial endovascular access is usually transfemoral (most common) or transbrachial (in cases of unfavorable VA-origin angle for the transfemoral approach). Recently, the transradial approach has been proposed [16,24]. Its advantages include easy hemostasis and comfort to the patient (the patient is able to sit and walk immediately after the procedure) [24]. The patient must have adequate ulnar arterial supply to the hand, so that occlusion of the radial artery will not result in an ischemic hand. Ulnar arterial supply is assessed before the procedure with the Allen test and possibly Doppler sonography.

After arterial access has been obtained and an appropriately sized arterial sheath secured in place, systemic heparinization is begun. According to our anticoagulation protocol, all patients are heparinized during the procedure with intravenous heparin, a 70–100 U/kg bolus followed by a 7–10 U/kg per hour infusion, with a goal of an activated clotting time of 250 to 300 seconds. Using a standard hydrophilic guide wire and a 6F guide catheter, the target subclavian artery is catheterized and the guide catheter advanced to just proximal to the VA (**Fig. 1**). The 6F guide catheter usually provides adequate stability. In cases of marked tortuosity of the subclavian artery or brachiocephalic trunk, an 80-cm 6F shuttle sheath may be necessary to provide a stable platform. If the brachiocephalic or subclavian arteries cannot be catheterized with the curved guide catheter, or if the shuttle sheath is necessary, the target brachiocephalic or subclavian artery is selected with a diagnostic catheter. Then, with the use of a 0.035-in exchange-length guide wire, the diagnostic catheter is removed and replaced with the guide catheter or shuttle sheath. This procedure requires some forethought because the groin or brachial sheath needs to be sized to allow placement of the guide catheter, or removed for placement of the long shuttle sheath. For further stability and better control, a 0.014-in or 0.018-in guide wire may be placed in the ipsilateral axillary artery through the side port to support the guide catheter and prevent it from moving (**Fig. 2**). After the guide catheter or sheath is stable in the subclavian artery, an angiogram is performed for quantification of the stenosis and measurement of the VA. The best view of the stenosis is then selected as a working projection. The degree of stenosis is determined in relation to the diameter of the normal segment of vessel immediately distal to the stenosis. Biplane road map images are then obtained and the stenosis is crossed with a curved-tip 0.014-in or 0.018-in guide wire. The curved tip helps to negotiate the stenosis and prevent subintimal dissection at the site of stenosis or distally within the VA. The wire tip is positioned in the distal cervical VA within the fluoroscopic field-of-view, providing additional stability to the system.

Angioplasty with a small balloon may be necessary in very tight stenoses to allow positioning of the definitive balloon stent system. Usually, we do not perform prestent angioplasty because most of the low-profile, balloon-mounted coronary stents can be navigated successfully across a tight stenosis without becoming dislodged from the angioplasty balloon. If prestent angioplasty is performed, pre- and postangioplasty neurologic examination is performed to assess possible procedural complications. A postangioplasty angiogram should also be performed to assess vessel injury (dissection, rupture, and emboli).

We have favored the use of balloon-expandable coronary stents to treat stenosis of vertebral origin because of accuracy in placement. Balloon-expandable coronary stents have a good combination of adequate radial force, low crossing profile, and limited foreshortening. Recently, we have begun to use drug-eluting stents (sirolimus coating), especially if the patient is diabetic (see **Figs. 1 and 2**). The expectation is a decrease in restenosis rates because the sirolimus inhibits smooth muscle and endothelial proliferation. Although experience described in the coronary literature largely supports such a practice [25,26], drug-eluting stents in cardiac procedures have been associated recently with clot formation in some cases, resulting in thrombosis at the stent site. We have not found this in noncardiac applications of the drug-eluting stents; however, we have continued antiplatelet therapy long term. Although we have used self-expanding stents, we reserve them for cases involving large vertebral arteries. The use of monorail or over-the-wire systems depends on the experience and comfort level of the operator.

The stent diameter is selected by considering the size of the normal segment of the VA immediately distal to the stenosis. VA-origin atherosclerotic lesions are usually focal, and accurate stent positioning is crucial. The stent length should be enough to extend proximally 1 mm to 2 mm into the lumen of the ipsilateral subclavian artery and at least 3 mm into the normal distal VA, covering the entire lesion.

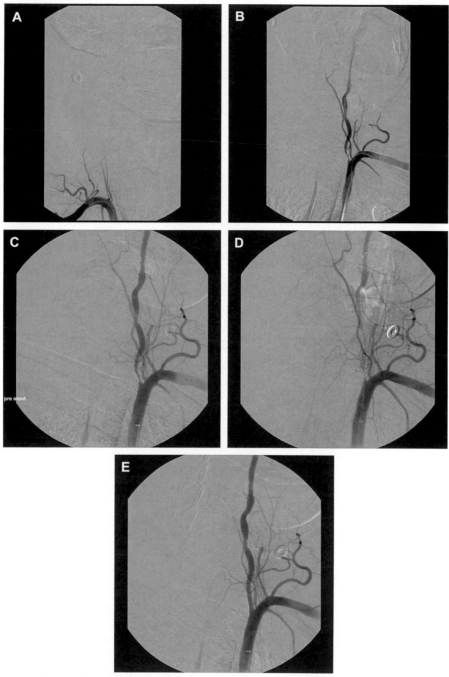

Fig. 1. A 52-year-old man with a history of diabetes and hypertension presented with recurrent posterior circulation symptoms. (*A*) Frontal right subclavian arteriogram shows no filling of the right VA. (*B*) Frontal left subclavian arteriogram shows a severe stenosis at the origin of the left VA. (*C*) A shuttle sheath has been placed in the proximal left subclavian artery in preparation for placement of the angioplasty balloon and stent. (*D*) Frontal left subclavian arteriogram demonstrates the positioning of a sirolimus-coated stent across the stenosis, which results in near occlusion of the left VA. (*E*) Frontal left subclavian arteriogram after the angioplasty and stent deployment shows restoration of the normal lumen.

The balloon-expandable stent is advanced and positioned. Before deployment, the nominal balloon and stent diameter, and the burst pressure of the balloon, are ascertained. The balloon is inflated under continuous fluoroscopic and road map guidance, to assure appropriate positioning and

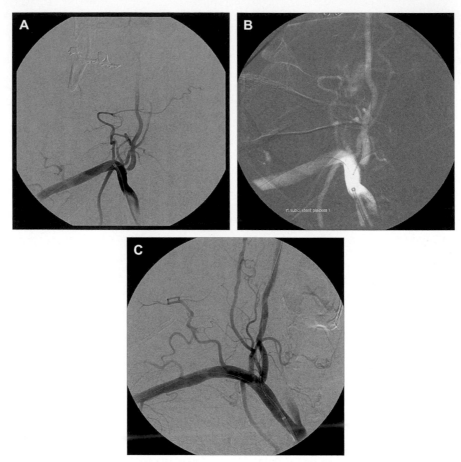

Fig. 2. A 63-year-old man with a history of diabetes presented with a visual field deficit and dizziness. Angiography (not shown) demonstrated that the left common carotid artery and the left subclavian arteries were occluded. (*A*) Frontal right subclavian arteriogram demonstrates a severe stenosis at the origin of the right VA (greater than 70%). (*B*) Road map image through the guide catheter demonstrates a 0.018-in guide wire in the right axillary artery for better support and stability, and positioning of the sirolimus stent across the stenosis. (*C*) Frontal right subclavian arteriogram after the angioplasty and stent deployment reveals restoration of the normal lumen in the right VA. The guide wires in the right VA and right axillary artery, and the guide catheter, can be identified.

complete stent expansion. An angiogram is performed in the working projection (used to deploy the stent) to document the technical result of the procedure (successful if less than 20% of residual stenosis). Final angiographic images of the intracranial posterior circulation are obtained to assess the flow to the vertebrobasilar system and any thromboembolic complications. The final angiogram is compared with the initial preprocedure angiogram. The patient's neurologic status is reassessed at the end of the procedure and, if unchanged, the heparin infusion is stopped. In our institution, the patient is continued on clopidogrel bisulfate, 75 mg a day for at least 3 months, and aspirin, 325 mg a day, for at least 6 months after the procedure. The patient is followed clinically, and if recurrent or new symptoms occur, a repeat angiogram is performed to assess restenosis.

Treatment of VA-origin stenosis in the left VA arising directly from the aorta or from the proximal subclavian artery requires a technique similar to that used for the brachiocephalic or subclavian artery treatments discussed later.

Discussion and long-term results

Based on published carotid data, patients who have vertebrobasilar ischemic symptoms are treated initially in most centers with antiplatelet agents, anticoagulants, or a combination of both (see Refs. [5–7,11,13,14]), even though, as noted earlier, the efficacy of this approach has not been established definitively. Persistent posterior circulation ischemic symptoms or events after antiplatelet or anticoagulant medication prompt alternatives. Surgical techniques for VA-origin disease include endarterectomy, vertebral reimplantation into either the subclavian or common carotid arteries, and bypass. Because of its complexity and technical difficulties, however, surgery for VA-origin disease is associated with an approximately 4% mortality and up to a 20% risk of procedural complications [5,7,11,13].

Percutaneous angioplasty has emerged as a reasonable alternative to open surgery [12,14]. Complications related to angioplasty (including dissection, occlusion, and thromboembolism) have been described in the pertinent literature, and the procedure is associated with an approximately 9% risk of transient neurologic deficits and up to a 15% restenosis rate [12,14,17,18]. Nevertheless, angioplasty generally is considered safe and is associated with symptomatic improvement [7,12,14].

The origin of the VA has a large amount of elastin and smooth muscle, resulting in elastic recoil following angioplasty, which can result in restenosis [4,5]. To overcome the elastic recoil and improve the long-term results, stenting was proposed. Multiple studies have shown that angioplasty and stenting of the VA origin is feasible, effective, safe, and associated with low periprocedural complication rates (see Refs. [4–8,10–16,19–22]). The procedure can be performed by different endovascular routes, including transfemoral (most common), transbrachial, and the recently described transradial [16,24]. Stent placement is believed to decrease the incidence of elastic recoil and restenosis and, in addition, it may protect against distal embolism by smoothing luminal irregularities, thereby decreasing flow turbulence in the origin of the vessel [7,10,12,14]. Our experience is comparable with the results in the pertinent literature demonstrating that angioplasty and stenting of the VA origin is safe, with a high technical success rate and improvement or resolution of symptoms after the procedure [27].

Resolution of symptoms following the procedure, frequency of restenosis, and recurrence of vertebrobasilar ischemic symptoms are crucial issues in the long-term results of the procedure. Furthermore, patient selection, clinical versus radiologic follow-up, and duration of follow-up all influence the long-term results [11].

The frequency of significant restenosis (greater than 50%) after stent placement varies greatly in published reports, ranging from 0% to 43% [4]. Arterial wall injury during angioplasty and stenting induces local inflammation and disorderly proliferation of smooth muscle cells, resulting in intimal hyperplasia and, subsequently, restenosis [15]. The tortuosity of the proximal VA may also be a determinant in restenosis, because the artificial straightening of this segment likely stresses the arterial wall [4]. The mechanical characteristics of stents and stent fracture are other potential factors associated with restenosis [6].

Albuquerque and colleagues [4] reported on 33 patients who had proximal VA disease and underwent angioplasty and stent deployment. The technical success rate was 97% (32 of 33). No symptomatic complications resulted from the procedures. Angiographic follow-up obtained in 30 patients revealed moderate-to-severe restenosis in 43.3% of these patients; however, the restenosis rate and recurrence of symptoms showed no correlation.

Chastain and colleagues [5] investigated the feasibility, safety, and outcome of angioplasty and stenting of the proximal VA in 50 patients and 55 vessels. The procedure was successful in 98% of the cases and no procedure-related complications were noted. Ninety percent of the patient population had angiographic follow-up at 6 months, which revealed significant restenosis in 10%. Clinical follow-up was performed in 49 patients at a mean of 25 months, with only 2 patients having neurologic symptoms.

Weber and colleagues [6] studied 38 patients who had symptomatic stenosis of VA origin that was stented. The technical success was 100%. Two patients had procedural dissections that were asymptomatic and one patient had worsening of symptoms after the procedure. At follow-up (mean 11 months), 23 of 26 patients were asymptomatic. Of the three symptomatic patients, only one had symptoms related to the vertebrobasilar system. The other two patients had unrelated atherosclerotic infarcts. Angiographically documented restenosis was seen in 10 of 26 patients, all of them asymptomatic. Two stents were occluded.

In the series published by Jenkins and colleagues [13], 38 vertebral arteries were treated in 32 patients, with procedural success achieved in all patients. One patient experienced a TIA 1 hour after the procedure. Thirty-one of thirty-two patients (97%) were asymptomatic at a mean follow-up of 10.6 months. The restenosis rate was 3%.

A study by Lin and colleagues [19] in which 80 symptomatic patients with 90 lesions were treated with balloon-expandable stents demonstrated a technical success rate of 100%. Periprocedural posterior and anterior circulation strokes occurred in 2.5% and 1.7%, respectively. The angiographic restenosis rate was 28% in 40 lesions, with a mean follow-up of 11.7 months. The rate of restenosis was influenced by the length of the original stenosis;

the rate was 21% in stenosis of less then 5 mm and 50% in lesions greater than 10 mm in length.

Eberhardt and colleagues [21] analyzed the published clinical data from more than 300 interventions for proximal VA stenosis and found a combined 0.3% risk of death, 0.7% risk of stroke, 5.5% risk of periprocedural neurologic complications, and 25.7% restenosis rate, with a mean follow-up of 11.8 months. The restenosis rate was not correlated to recurrence of symptoms.

Other, smaller series have shown high technical success rates and low rates of procedural complications [8,12]. In the series reported by Piotin and colleagues [14], seven lesions in seven patients were treated successfully. No perioperative complications were noted. Clinical follow-up showed immediate resolution or improvement of symptoms in all cases. One patient had recurrent symptoms but no evidence of restenosis. All other patients had no sonographic evidence of restenosis.

Some recent studies have explored the use of protection devices to preclude embolization during angioplasty and stenting of VA origin. Qureshi and colleagues [20] treated 12 patients using distal protection devices; they had technical success in 11 patients (primary technical end point), and no stroke or death was observed at 1-month follow-up (primary clinical end point). This study demonstrated that angioplasty and stenting of the VA origin using distal protection devices is feasible and safe. Wehman and colleagues [11] recommended the use of distal protection devices in larger vertebral arteries (diameter greater than 3.5 mm), in cases that have a favorable angle of the VA origin, and in the treatment of ulcerated lesions. Widespread use of protection devices awaits further study on their efficacy.

In our experience with 25 patients, the contralateral VA was occluded, hypoplastic, absent, or had greater than 50% stenosis in 23. Thirteen of twenty-five patients demonstrated angiographic evidence of significant anterior circulation disease. In 18 of the 25 patients, the left VA was affected, with a mean stenosis of 83%. In these 25 patients, 28 procedures were performed; 23 were angioplasty and stenting and 5 were angioplasty alone. The technical success (stenosis reduced to less than 20%) was achieved in 26 of the 28 procedures (93%). No procedure-related TIA, stroke, or death occurred. Nineteen of twenty-five patients had a mean follow-up of 24 months. Five of the nineteen had recurrent symptoms of vertebrobasilar ischemia, and three patients were re-treated.

In summary, angioplasty and stenting of the VA origin in patients presenting with medically refractory vertebrobasilar insufficiency symptoms is feasible, safe, and effective, with significant improvement of symptoms.

Considerations for endovascular treatment of the innominate and subclavian arteries

Innominate and subclavian artery stenosis is found frequently in patients who have multivessel vascular disease, and they account for up to 17% of patients presenting with neurologic symptoms due to extracranial vascular disease [28–30]. Of patients who have occlusive disease of the innominate or subclavian artery, approximately 50% have concomitant coronary artery disease, 27% have peripheral vascular disease, and 29% have carotid/vertebral disease [29,31]. Occlusive disease of these vessels occurs in relatively younger patients, when compared with other types of atherosclerotic diseases, with a slight male predominance [29].

Atherosclerosis is, by far, the most common cause of occlusive disease in the innominate and subclavian arteries, followed by Takayasu's arteritis, fibromuscular dysplasia, trauma, thoracic outlet syndrome, and radiation-induced stenosis [28,29].

Innominate and subclavian artery stenting became an accepted therapeutic tool during the 1990s. Its major role was to treat unsuccessful angioplasties and improve long-term postprocedural patency of the vessels treated [29,31]. Its definitive role and its indications, however, are not completely clear [28,32]. As with the endovascular treatment of the VA origin, most of the available data about angioplasty and stenting of the innominate and subclavian artery are in the form of retrospective case series [29].

Clinical aspects

When they are symptomatic neurologically, innominate lesions may present with anterior circulation symptoms (due to symptoms referred to the right carotid system), posterior circulation symptoms (through the right VA), or both. Cherry and colleagues [33] reported that 50% of their patients had anterior circulation symptoms, 40% had posterior circulation symptoms, and 10% had both.

Although subclavian artery stenosis might be asymptomatic because of the rich collateral vascular network, neurologic symptoms of vertebrobasilar ischemia may occur [10,29,31]. Stenosis of the subclavian artery can decrease the flow to the ipsilateral VA, or even reverse the flow with subclavian steal (Fig. 3) [10].

Both innominate and subclavian artery stenosis may present with symptoms and signs of upper limb ischemia, including claudication and digital emboli [29].

All patients should have a complete history elicited and a physical and neurologic examination. Cervical bruits, blood pressure difference in the arms, and finger ulcers are all signs of innominate

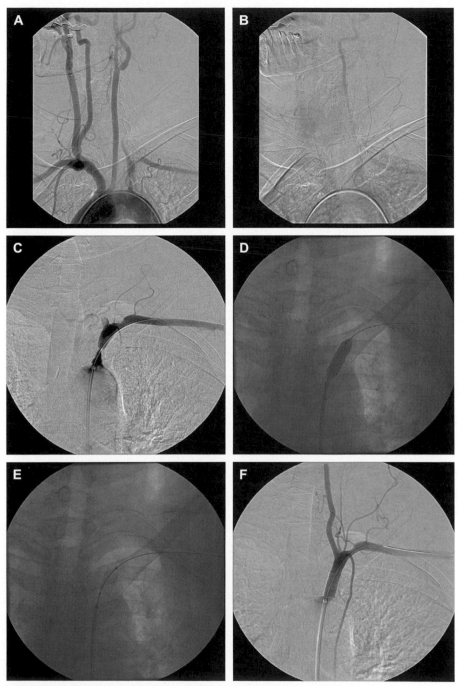

Fig. 3. A 54-year-old woman with a history of peripheral vascular disease presented with dizziness. (*A*) Left anterior oblique aortic arch projection, demonstrating a large right VA and a high-grade stenosis in the proximal left subclavian artery and minimal antegrade flow in the left VA. (*B*) Later phase of the aortic arch injection, demonstrating retrograde filling of the VA and faint filling of the left subclavian artery, indicating subclavian steal. (*C*) Frontal left subclavian arteriogram performed with the guide catheter at the origin of the left subclavian artery, demonstrating the high-grade stenosis in the proximal subclavian artery, minimal antegrade flow in the left VA, and another 50% stenosis in the left subclavian artery distal to the left VA. (*D*) Frontal view with the angioplasty balloon inflated across the proximal left subclavian stenosis. (*E*) Frontal view of the expanded stent in the proximal left subclavian stenosis. (*F*) Frontal left subclavian arteriogram through the guide catheter after the angioplasty, demonstrating placement of the stent. The normal lumen of the proximal left subclavian artery has been restored and antegrade flow in the left VA has been preserved. With the increased flow in the left subclavian artery, the more distal stenosis does not seem to be quite as severe. The guide wire and guide catheter remain in place.

or subclavian artery stenosis [29]. Gadolinium-MR angiography, CT angiography, and digital subtraction angiograms should be used to confirm the diagnosis and plan treatment.

Indications for treatment

Indications for treatment are

Signs and symptoms of vertebrobasilar ischemia
Signs and symptoms of upper extremity ischemia
Signs and symptoms in territories supplied by grafts (eg, leg claudication in patients with axillofemoral grafts)

Technical aspects and results

Most of the principles described earlier for angioplasty and stenting of the VA origin also apply to the endovascular treatment of the innominate or subclavian arteries. Our pre-, intra- and postprocedure medication regimen is also the same. A complete cervicocranial angiogram should be performed for assessment of the cerebral circulation and collateral pathways. Although the brachial or radial approaches are attractive, they may be difficult because of the more proximal stenosis eliminating the palpable pulse. Ultrasound localization can be helpful in these instances.

With the transfemoral approach, the guide catheter is positioned frequently in the aorta or at the origin of the desired vessel for proximal lesions. Road map images are acquired from this location. Catheterization of the brachiocephalic or subclavian artery may require use of a 4F diagnostic catheter through the larger guide catheter or sheath. The diagnostic catheter must be longer than the guide catheter or sheath. A 0.014-in guide wire for the angioplasty balloon and stent is placed across the stenosis, well into the axillary artery, and the diagnostic catheter removed. Appropriately sized sheaths, guide catheters, balloons, and stents must be chosen to avoid size mismatches in selected materials, which can increase the complexity of the procedure. Although no data prove that procedural variations lessen procedural success and increase complications, it seems reasonable to assume that this is the case.

Usually, balloon-expandable stents are used and should cover the entire stenotic segment (see Fig. 3). As in the carotid or vertebral system, balloon-expandable stents are used only when the site is not subject to movement, because collapse of a balloon-expandable stent can be catastrophic. In long-segment stenoses (greater then 4.0 cm), self-expanding stents should be used [31]. Significant protrusion of the stent into the aortic arch or common carotid artery origin and covering the VA origin should be avoided if possible because these

stent locations may increase the risk of vessel occlusion or embolization [29].

In cases of associated VA-origin and subclavian artery stenosis, the "kissing balloon" technique can be used. For this technique, two microwires are advanced through a femoral approach. One wire is used to catheterize the VA origin and a coronary balloon is positioned across the stenosis. The other wire is advanced through the subclavian artery and positioned across the stenosis. Then, both balloons are inflated simultaneously [7]. The double-balloon technique also can be used. Through a radial or brachial approach, a microwire is used to select the VA origin, and the angioplasty balloon is positioned and inflated at the stenosis. Through a femoral approach, the stenotic lesion at the subclavian artery is crossed and angioplasty is performed. After angioplasty of the subclavian artery, the VA balloon is deflated. This technique is useful to protect the vertebrobasilar system from potential embolization from the subclavian artery angioplasty [34]. The decision of whether or not these segments will be stented depends on the results of the angioplasty.

Huttl and colleagues [35] retrospectively assessed the success of percutaneous transluminal angioplasty (PTA) in treating innominate artery stenoses and occlusions in a large series. In symptomatic patients (upper limb claudication, TIA, vertebrobasilar insufficiency) with significant stenosis (>60%), innominate artery PTA was performed. The primary success rate was 96.4%. Complications included one left occipital lobe infarction (2%), two puncture-site thromboses (3%), and four TIAs (6%). Two patients who had restenosis were treated successfully with repeated PTA. Cumulative primary patency was 98% at 6 months and 93% at 16 to 117 months; secondary patency was 100% at 6 months and 98% at 12 to 117 months. Sixty-one percent of the patients became asymptomatic, 32% improved, and 7% showed no improvement. The investigators concluded that angioplasty of the innominate artery is safe and effective and that for innominate artery stenosis and short occlusion, PTA should be the treatment of choice [35].

The technical and clinical success rates of endovascular treatment of subclavian artery stenosis are similarly high [28,31,36,37]. Complications range from 0% to approximately 10% [28,29,31,37].

Brountzos and colleagues [31] reviewed the immediate and midterm results of primary stenting for innominate and subclavian artery occlusive lesions in a series of 48 patients who had serious comorbid conditions. Technical success was achieved in 96%, and clinical success in 94% of the patients. Four complications were reported (two puncture site hematomas, one distal hand embolization, and one cerebral TIA). Two patients died from other causes within 30 days, and seven patients were lost to follow-up. Mean follow-up was 16.7 months. Five patients had recurrent lesions. The cumulative primary patency rates were 91.7% and 77% at 12 and 24 months, respectively. Secondary patency rates were 96.5% and 91.7% at 12 and 24 months, respectively [31].

Amor and colleagues reported their experience with 89 subclavian obstructive lesions treated with stenting: 76 (85.3%) stenoses and 13 (14.6%) total occlusions [28]. Technical success was obtained in 83 (93.3%) (100% in stenotic lesions and 53.8% in total occlusions). Nine global complications (10.1%) included five (5.6%) at the site of puncture, two (2.2%) distal embolizations, and two (2.3%) major events. The long-term mean follow-up was 3.51 years, during which time 13 (16.8%) restenoses and 2 (2.6%) reocclusions were noted. Subgroup analysis of patients who had stenting after predilatation versus direct stenting techniques showed in-hospital complications only in the first group, with a restenosis rate of 28.5% versus 4.7%, respectively [28].

Al-Mubarak studied a series of 38 patients, with technical and clinical success achieved in 35 patients. They concluded that stenting for subclavian artery occlusive disease has favorable immediate and late (follow-up 20 ± 4 months) clinical outcomes and may be considered as a primary therapy [36]. Bates and colleagues [37] reported on a series of 101 stents placed in 91 patients, with a 72% 5-year patency rate, and drew a similar conclusion.

Henry and colleagues [38] compared the long-term results of subclavian artery angioplasty with and without stent placement. They reported an overall technical success rate of 91% and a 2.6% procedural complication rate (complications included a TIA, a fatal stroke, and an arterial thrombosis 24 hours after the procedure). The combined 8-year primary and secondary patency rates were 83% and 90%, respectively. No significant differences were noted between the two groups, however, and the investigators concluded that stents do not seem to improve long-term patency.

Our series of 11 patients who underwent treatment for subclavian artery stenosis resulted in no TIAs or strokes. One patient had bilateral subclavian artery stenosis, which was treated with angioplasty and stenting. Six self-expanding and two balloon-expandable stents were used. The patients who had angioplasty alone were observed for 1 hour during the procedure to assure subclavian artery patency and absence of intimal tear, clot formation, and recurrent (rebound) stenosis. In summary, patients presenting with symptoms due to stenosis of the innominate or subclavian arteries seem to benefit from the endovascular treatment of these lesions.

References

[1] Moufarrij NA, Little JR, Furlan AJ, et al. VA stenosis: long-term follow-up. Stroke 1984;15(2):260–3.

[2] Wityk RJ, Chang HM, Rosengart A, et al. Proximal extracranial VA disease in the New England medical center posterior circulation registry. Arch Neurol 1998;55(4):470–8.

[3] Caplan LR, Wityk RJ, Glass TA, et al. New England medical center posterior circulation registry. Ann Neurol 2004;56(3):389–98.

[4] Albuquerque FC, Fiorella D, Han P, et al. A reappraisal of angioplasty and stenting for the treatment of vertebral origin stenosis. Neurosurgery 2003;53(3):607–14.

[5] Chastain HD 2nd, Campbell MS, Iyer S, et al. Extracranial VA stent placement: in-hospital and follow-up results. J Neurosurg 1999;91(4): 547–52.

[6] Weber W, Mayer TE, Henkes H, et al. Efficacy of stent angioplasty for symptomatic stenoses of the proximal VA. Eur J Radiol 2005;56(2):240–7.

[7] Henry M, Henry I, Klonaris C, et al. Percutaneous transluminal angioplasty and stenting of extracranial VA stenosis. In: Henry M, Ohki T, Polydorou A, et al, editors. Angioplasty and stenting of the carotid and supra-aortic trunks. 1st edition. London (UK): Taylor and Francis Medicine; 2003. p. 673–82.

[8] Cloud GC, Crawley F, Clifton A, et al. VA origin angioplasty and primary stenting: safety and restenosis rates in a prospective series. J Neurol Neurosurg Psychiatr 2003;74(5):586–90.

[9] Amin-Hanjani S, Du X, Zhao M, et al. Use of quantitative magnetic resonance angiography to stratify stroke risk in symptomatic vertebrobasilar disease. Stroke 2005;36(6):1140–5.

[10] Malek AM, Higashida RT, Phatouros CC, et al. Treatment of posterior circulation ischemia with extracranial percutaneous balloon angioplasty and stent placement. Stroke 1999;30(10): 2073–85.

[11] Wehman JC, Hanel RA, Guidot CA, et al. Atherosclerotic occlusive extracranial VA disease: indications for intervention, endovascular techniques, short-term and long-term results. J Interv Cardiol 2004;17(4):219–32.

[12] Hauth EA, Gissler HM, Drescher R, et al. Angioplasty or stenting of extra- and intracranial VA stenoses. Cardiovasc Intervent Radiol 2004; 27(1):51–7.

[13] Jenkins JS, White CJ, Ramee SR, et al. VA stenting. Catheter Cardiovasc Interv 2001;54(1):1–5.

[14] Piotin M, Spelle L, Martin JB, et al. Percutaneous transluminal angioplasty and stenting of the proximal VA for symptomatic stenosis. AJNR Am J Neuroradiol 2000;21(4):727–31.

[15] Hayashi K, Kitagawa N, Morikawa M, et al. A case of intimal hyperplasia induced by stenting for VA origin stenosis: assessed on intravascular ultrasound. Neurol Res 2003;25(4):357–60.

[16] Fessler RD, Wakhloo AK, Lanzino G, et al. Transradial approach for VA stenting: technical case report. Neurosurgery 2000;46(6):1524–7.

[17] Higashida RT, Tsai FY, Halbach VV, et al. Transluminal angioplasty for atherosclerotic disease of the vertebral and basilar arteries. J Neurosurg 1993;78(2):192–8.

[18] Bruckmann H, Ringelstein EB, Buchner H, et al. Percutaneous transluminal angioplasty of the VA. A therapeutic alternative to operative reconstruction of proximal VA stenoses. J Neurol 1986;233(6):336–9.

[19] Lin YH, Liu YC, Tseng WYI, et al. The impact of lesion length on angiographic restenosis after VA origin stenting. Eur J Vasc Endovasc Surg 2006; 32(4):379–85.

[20] Qureshi AI, Kirmani JF, Harris-Lane P, et al. VA origin stent placement with distal protection: technical and clinical results. AJNR Am J Neuroradiol 2006;27(5):1140–5.

[21] Eberhardt O, Naegele T, Raygrotzki S, et al. Stenting of vertebrobasilar arteries in symptomatic atherosclerotic disease and acute occlusion: case series and review of the literature. J Vasc Surg 2006;43(6):1145–54.

[22] Lin YH, Juang JM, Jeng JS, et al. Symptomatic ostial VA stenosis treated with tubular coronary stents: clinical results and restenosis analysis. J Endovasc Ther 2004;11(6):719–26.

[23] Huber P. Cerebral arteries: VA. In: Cerebral angiography. 2nd edition. New York: Thieme; 1982. p. 136–40.

[24] Layton KF, Kallmes DF, Cloft HJ. The radial artery access site for interventional neuroradiology procedures. AJNR Am J Neuroradiol 2006;27(5): 1151–4.

[25] Abizaid A, Costa MA, Blanchard D, et al. Sirolimus-eluting stents inhibit neointimal hyperplasia in diabetic patients. Insights from the RAVEL Trial. Eur Heart J 2004;25(2):107–12.

[26] Regar E, Serruys PW, Bode C, et al. Angiographic findings of the multicenter randomized study with the sirolimus-eluting Bx velocity balloon-expandable stent (RAVEL): sirolimus-eluting stents inhibit restenosis irrespective of the vessel size. Circulation 2002;106(15):1949–56.

[27] Dabus G, Gerstle RJ, Derdeyn CP, et al. Endovascular treatment of the vertebral artery origin in patients with symptoms of vertebrobasilar ischemia. Neuroradiology 2006;48:917–23.

[28] Amor M, Eid-Lidt G, Chati Z, et al. Endovascular treatment of the subclavian artery: stent implantation with or without predilatation. Catheter Cardiovasc Interv 2004;63(3):364–70.

[29] Brountzos EN, Malagari K, Kelekis DA. Endovascular treatment of occlusive lesions of the subclavian and innominate arteries. Cardiovasc Intervent Radiol 2006;29(4):503–10.

[30] Kandarpa K, Becker GJ, Hunink MG, et al. Transcatheter interventions for the treatment of peripheral atherosclerotic lesions: part I. J Vasc Interv Radiol 2001;12(6):683–95.

[31] Brountzos EN, Petersen B, Binkert C, et al. Primary stenting of subclavian and innominate artery occlusive disease: a single center's experience. Cardiovasc Intervent Radiol 2004;27(6): 616–23.

[32] Society of Interventional Radiology Standards of Practice Committee. Guidelines for percutaneous transluminal angioplasty. J Vasc Interv Radiol 2003;14:209S–17S.

[33] Cherry KJ Jr, McCullough JL, Hallett JW Jr, et al. Technical principles of direct innominate artery revascularization: a comparison of endarterectomy and bypass grafts. J Vasc Surg 1989;9(5): 718–23.

[34] Staikov IN, Do DD, Remonda L, et al. The site of atheromatosis in the subclavian and vertebral arteries and its implication for angioplasty. Neuroradiology 1999;41(7):537–42.

[35] Huttl K, Nemes B, Simonffy A, et al. Angioplasty of the innominate artery in 89 patients: experience over 19 years. Cardiovasc Intervent Radiol 2002;25(2):109–14.

[36] Al-Mubarak N, Liu MW, Dean LS, et al. Immediate and late outcomes of subclavian artery stenting. Catheter Cardiovasc Interv 1999;46(2): 169–72.

[37] Bates MC, Broce M, Lavigne PS, et al. Subclavian artery stenting: factors influencing long-term outcome. Catheter Cardiovasc Interv 2004; 61(1):5–11.

[38] Henry M, Amor M, Henry I, et al. Percutaneous transluminal angioplasty of the subclavian arteries. J Endovasc Surg 1999;6(1): 33–41.

ELSEVIER
SAUNDERS

NEUROIMAGING
CLINICS
OF NORTH AMERICA

Neuroimag Clin N Am 17 (2007) 393–395

Index

Note: Page numbers of article titles are in **boldface** type.

neuroimaging.theclinics.com

doi:10.1016/S1052-5149(07)00079-2

B

C

E

F

G

H

Moving?

Make sure your subscription moves with you!

To notify us of your new address, find your **Clinics Account Number** (located on your mailing label above your name), and contact customer service at:

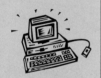

E-mail: elspcs@elsevier.com

800-654-2452 (subscribers in the U.S. & Canada)
407-345-4000 (subscribers outside of the U.S. & Canada)

Fax number: 407-363-9661

Elsevier Periodicals Customer Service
6277 Sea Harbor Drive
Orlando, FL 32887-4800

*To ensure uninterrupted delivery of your subscription, please notify us at least 4 weeks in advance of move.

ELSEVIER